The Healing Journey: Discovering Mental Health and Wellbeing

Kava

The Healing Journey: Discovering Mental Health and Wellbeing

Copyright © 2023 by Kava

All rights reserved. No part of this book may be reproduced or transmitted in any form or by any means, electronic or mechanical, including photocopying, recording, or by any information storage and retrieval system, without permission in writing from the publisher.

This book is a work of fiction. Names, characters, places, and incidents either are the product of the author's imagination or are used fictitiously. Any resemblance to actual events, locales, persons, living or dead, is entirely coincidental.

The first edition was published in 2023

ISBN:
Published by:
Sunshine
1663 Liberty Drive
Hyderabad, IN 47403
www.Sunshinepublishers.com

This book is self-published using on-demand printing and publishing, which allows it to be printed and distributed globally

TABLE OF CONTENT

Chapter 1: Understanding Mental Health   08

The Importance of Mental Health

Common Mental Health Disorders

Factors Influencing Mental Health

Stigma Surrounding Mental Illness

Chapter 2: Exploring Wellbeing   17

Defining Wellbeing

Physical Wellbeing

Emotional Wellbeing

Social Wellbeing

Spiritual Wellbeing

Chapter 3: The Mind-Body Connection — 28

Understanding the Mind-Body Connection

Effects of Stress on Mental Health

Techniques for Managing Stress

The Role of Sleep in Mental Wellbeing

Chapter 4: Nurturing Positive Relationships — 36

The Power of Relationships

Building Healthy Communication

Resolving Conflict

Boundaries in Relationships

Chapter 5: Developing Self-Awareness — 44

The Importance of Self-Awareness

Exploring Personal Values

Identifying Strengths and Weaknesses

Practicing Self-Compassion

Chapter 6: Cultivating Resilience　　52

Understanding Resilience

Strategies for Building Resilience

Overcoming Adversity

Embracing Change

Chapter 7: Seeking Help and Support　　60

Recognizing When to Seek Help

Types of Mental Health Professionals

Therapy Options

Support Networks and Resources

Chapter 8: Lifestyle Factors for Mental Wellbeing   69

Diet and Nutrition

Regular Exercise and Physical Activity

Mindfulness and Meditation

Hobbies and Leisure Activities

Chapter 9: Promoting Mental Health in the Workplace   77

The Importance of Mental Health at Work

Creating a Supportive Work Environment

Reducing Work-Related Stress

Employee Assistance Programs

Chapter 10: Maintaining Mental Health in the Digital Age   85

The Impact of Technology on Mental Health

Establishing Healthy Technology Habits

Managing Social Media and Online Presence

Balancing Screen Time and Real-Life Connections

Chapter 11: Embracing a Holistic Approach to Mental Wellbeing   93

Integrating Mind, Body, and Spirit

Incorporating Alternative Therapies

Exploring Holistic Practices

Finding Balance in Daily Life

Chapter 12: The Journey Towards Mental Health and Wellbeing   101

Embracing the Healing Journey

Setting Personal Goals

Celebrating Progress and Success

Sustaining Mental Health and Wellbeing

Conclusion: A Lifetime of Mental Health and Wellbeing   109

Chapter 1: Understanding Mental Health

The Importance of Mental Health

In today's fast-paced and demanding world, it is crucial to recognize the importance of mental health. Mental health is an integral part of our overall well-being, affecting how we think, feel, and act. It plays a significant role in our ability to cope with stress, build meaningful relationships, and achieve personal fulfillment. As such, understanding and prioritizing mental health is essential for everyone, regardless of age, gender, or background.

Public health initiatives have increasingly highlighted the significance of mental health as a vital component of overall wellness. Just as physical health is acknowledged and addressed, mental health deserves the same attention and care. The impact of mental health on individuals, families, communities, and society as a whole cannot be overstated.

When mental health is neglected, the consequences can be detrimental. Mental health disorders, such as depression, anxiety, and bipolar disorder, can significantly impair an individual's quality of life. They can hinder daily functioning, disrupt relationships, and lead to a sense of hopelessness. By recognizing the importance of mental health, we can take proactive steps to prevent and address these conditions.

Moreover, mental health is closely intertwined with physical health. The mind and body are interconnected, and one's mental state can directly impact their physical well-being. Stress, for instance, can manifest as physical symptoms. By prioritizing mental health, we not only enhance our emotional resilience but also promote overall physical health and longevity.

In recent years, society has made strides in reducing the stigma surrounding mental health. However, there is still work to be done. By educating ourselves and others about mental health, we can break down barriers and foster a more inclusive and compassionate society. Understanding the importance of mental health allows us to support and advocate for those struggling with mental health issues, promoting their well-being and access to appropriate care.

In conclusion, the importance of mental health cannot be emphasized enough. It is an integral part of our overall well-being and directly affects our ability to lead fulfilling lives. By recognizing mental health as a vital component of public health, we can prioritize its promotion and prevention. Through education, understanding, and support, we can create a society that values and prioritizes mental health, benefiting individuals and communities alike. Let us embark on this journey towards mental health and well-being together, ensuring a brighter and healthier future for all.

Common Mental Health Disorders

In today's fast-paced and demanding world, mental health has become a pressing concern for people from all walks of life. The prevalence of mental health disorders has risen dramatically, affecting individuals, families, and communities across the globe. This subchapter aims to shed light on some of the most common mental health disorders, providing a comprehensive understanding of their symptoms, causes, and available treatments.

1. Anxiety Disorders: Anxiety disorders, such as generalized anxiety disorder, social anxiety disorder, and panic disorder, are characterized by excessive worry, fear, and unease. These disorders can significantly impact a person's ability to function in daily life, often leading to avoidance behaviors.

2. Depression: Depression is a mood disorder that causes persistent feelings of sadness, hopelessness, and a loss of interest in activities. It affects millions of people worldwide and can lead to severe emotional and physical distress if left untreated.

3. Bipolar Disorder: Bipolar disorder is a condition marked by extreme mood swings, ranging from manic episodes of elevated energy and euphoria to depressive episodes of profound sadness and despair. These mood swings can disrupt daily life and impair relationships.

4. Eating Disorders: Eating disorders, such as anorexia nervosa, bulimia nervosa, and binge eating disorder, are characterized by unhealthy relationships with food and body image. They can have severe physical and psychological consequences if not addressed promptly.

5. Post-Traumatic Stress Disorder (PTSD): PTSD is a disorder that can develop after experiencing or witnessing a traumatic event. Individuals with PTSD may experience flashbacks, nightmares, and intense anxiety, often leading to avoidance of triggers associated with the traumatic event.

6. Substance Use Disorders: Substance use disorders involve the misuse or addiction to substances such as drugs or alcohol. They can have devastating effects on an individual's physical and mental health, as well as their relationships and overall functioning.

Understanding these common mental health disorders is crucial for promoting mental health and wellbeing in public health. By recognizing the signs and symptoms of these disorders, individuals can seek appropriate support and treatment. It is important to remember that mental health disorders are not a personal weakness but rather medical conditions that require professional help.

If you or someone you know is struggling with any of these disorders, it is essential to seek help from mental health professionals. Treatment options may include therapy, medication, lifestyle changes, and support groups. With the right support and treatment, individuals can manage their symptoms, improve their quality of life, and achieve mental wellbeing.

Remember, mental health matters, and seeking help is a sign of strength. Let us work together to create a society that values and promotes mental health for all.

Factors Influencing Mental Health

Mental health is a crucial aspect of overall wellbeing, and understanding the factors that influence it is essential for achieving and maintaining a healthy mind. In this subchapter, we will explore some of the key factors that can significantly impact our mental health and wellbeing.

1. Biological Factors: Our genetics play a vital role in shaping our mental health. Certain inherited traits can make individuals more susceptible to mental health disorders such as depression, anxiety, or bipolar disorder. Additionally, imbalances in brain chemicals, known as neurotransmitters, can also contribute to the development of mental health conditions.

2. Environmental Factors: Our surroundings have a profound impact on our mental health. Factors such as living conditions, exposure to violence or trauma, access to healthcare, and socioeconomic status can significantly influence our mental wellbeing. Stressful life events, such as the loss of a loved one, divorce, or financial difficulties, can also impact our mental health.

3. Social Factors: Our social connections and support networks play a crucial role in promoting good mental health. Positive relationships with family, friends, and communities can provide emotional support, a sense of belonging, and opportunities for engagement and growth. On the other hand, social isolation, discrimination, and bullying can have detrimental effects on mental health.

4. Lifestyle Factors: Our lifestyle choices can greatly impact our mental wellbeing. Regular exercise, a balanced diet, and sufficient sleep are

essential for maintaining good mental health. Substance abuse, including excessive alcohol consumption or drug use, can significantly increase the risk of developing mental health disorders.

5. Psychological Factors: Our thoughts, emotions, and behaviors also play a significant role in our mental health. Negative thought patterns, such as pessimism or self-criticism, can contribute to the development of mental health conditions. Additionally, poor coping skills, low self-esteem, and unresolved trauma can also negatively impact mental wellbeing.

It is essential to recognize that mental health is influenced by a complex interplay of various factors, and no single factor can fully determine one's mental wellbeing. However, by understanding and addressing these factors, individuals can take proactive steps towards promoting their mental health and seeking appropriate support when needed.

In conclusion, mental health is influenced by a combination of biological, environmental, social, lifestyle, and psychological factors. By recognizing and understanding these factors, we can work towards creating environments and lifestyles that support good mental health for ourselves and for others.

Stigma Surrounding Mental Illness

In today's society, mental illness is a prevalent issue that affects individuals from all walks of life. However, despite its widespread occurrence, there remains a significant stigma surrounding mental health conditions. This subchapter aims to shed light on the negative perceptions and misconceptions associated with mental illness, while also emphasizing the importance of combating stigma for the sake of public health.

Stigma surrounding mental illness refers to the negative attitudes, beliefs, and stereotypes that society holds towards people with mental health conditions. These attitudes can result in discrimination and prejudice, leading to individuals feeling isolated, ashamed, and hesitant to seek help. The consequences of stigma are far-reaching, impacting both the individual's wellbeing and the overall public health.

One of the main reasons behind the stigma surrounding mental illness is a lack of understanding and awareness. Misconceptions about mental health conditions often lead to fear and ignorance, perpetuating the stigma further. It is essential to educate ourselves and others about mental health to dispel these misconceptions and foster empathy and support.

Another factor contributing to stigma is the portrayal of mental illness in popular media. Movies, television shows, and news outlets often depict individuals with mental health conditions as dangerous or unpredictable. These portrayals only serve to reinforce stereotypes and create a climate of fear and misunderstanding. Media representation must be more responsible and accurate to help reduce the stigma associated with mental illness.

The impact of stigma on public health cannot be overstated. When individuals feel stigmatized, they are less likely to seek help or adhere to treatment. This can lead to the worsening of symptoms, deterioration in overall health, and reduced quality of life. Additionally, stigma prevents open dialogue about mental health, making it difficult to implement effective prevention and intervention strategies.

To combat stigma surrounding mental illness, we must promote acceptance, understanding, and empathy. It is crucial to foster an environment where individuals can openly discuss their mental health without fear of judgment or discrimination. This can be achieved through community education programs, media campaigns, and policy changes that prioritize mental health awareness and destigmatization.

By challenging the stigma surrounding mental illness, we can create a society that supports and empowers individuals to seek help when needed. Through increased awareness and understanding, we can work towards a future where mental health is treated with the same importance as physical health. It is only by breaking down these barriers that we can truly achieve mental health and wellbeing for all.

In conclusion, the stigma surrounding mental illness is a significant barrier to public health. By addressing and challenging this stigma, we can create a more inclusive and supportive society for individuals living with mental health conditions. It is our collective responsibility to educate ourselves and others, promote empathy and understanding, and ensure that mental health is prioritized alongside physical health. Together, we can embark on a healing journey towards mental health and wellbeing for everyone.

Chapter 2: Exploring Wellbeing

Defining Wellbeing

In today's fast-paced and demanding world, it is becoming increasingly important to prioritize our mental health and wellbeing. But what exactly does "wellbeing" mean? How can we define it in a way that resonates with everyone, particularly those interested in public health? In this subchapter, we will explore the multifaceted concept of wellbeing and shed light on its significance for individuals and communities.

Wellbeing goes beyond the absence of illness; it encompasses a holistic state of being that includes physical, mental, and emotional health. It is a dynamic process that fluctuates throughout our lives, influenced by various factors such as our environment, relationships, and personal experiences. Wellbeing is not a destination but a continuous journey towards optimal health and happiness.

From a public health perspective, wellbeing extends beyond individual health and encompasses the overall health and happiness of communities. It is about creating an environment that promotes positive mental health and fosters social connections. Public health initiatives aimed at improving wellbeing focus on preventive measures, education, and the development of supportive systems and policies.

Understanding the dimensions of wellbeing helps us grasp its complexity. Physical wellbeing involves taking care of our bodies through regular exercise, balanced nutrition, and sufficient rest.

Mental wellbeing refers to our cognitive and emotional health, including our ability to cope with stress, manage emotions, and maintain a positive mindset. Emotional wellbeing involves recognizing and expressing our feelings in a healthy way, as well as cultivating resilience and self-compassion.

Social wellbeing emphasizes the significance of relationships and social connections in our lives. It includes having a supportive network of family, friends, and community, as well as feeling a sense of belonging and inclusion. Environmental wellbeing highlights the impact of our surroundings on our overall health, emphasizing the importance of living in a clean and sustainable environment.

Achieving wellbeing requires a proactive approach. It involves practicing self-care, setting boundaries, and prioritizing activities that bring joy and fulfillment. Cultivating mindfulness and engaging in activities that promote relaxation and stress reduction, such as meditation or spending time in nature, can also contribute to overall wellbeing.

Ultimately, wellbeing is a deeply personal and subjective experience. What brings wellbeing to one person may differ from another. However, by understanding the multidimensional nature of wellbeing and acknowledging its significance in public health, we can create a society that values and supports the mental health and wellbeing of all its members.

In the following chapters, we will delve deeper into specific strategies and practices that can enhance wellbeing, providing readers with practical tools to embark on their healing journey towards mental health and overall wellbeing.

Physical Wellbeing

In today's fast-paced world, it is easy to neglect our physical health. We often find ourselves consumed by work, stress, and the never-ending demands of our daily lives. However, achieving and maintaining physical wellbeing is essential for overall health and happiness. In this subchapter, we will explore the importance of physical wellbeing and discuss practical strategies to help you improve and maintain it.

Physical wellbeing encompasses various aspects, including nutrition, exercise, sleep, and self-care. It involves nourishing our bodies with the right foods, engaging in regular physical activity, getting sufficient rest, and taking care of ourselves both mentally and physically.

Proper nutrition plays a vital role in physical wellbeing. Consuming a balanced diet rich in fruits, vegetables, whole grains, and lean proteins provides our bodies with essential nutrients, vitamins, and minerals. It fuels our energy levels, improves our immune system, and promotes overall wellbeing. We will delve into the importance of nutrition and provide practical tips for adopting a healthy eating plan.

Regular exercise is another key component of physical wellbeing. Engaging in physical activity not only helps us maintain a healthy weight but also reduces the risk of chronic diseases, improves cardiovascular health, and boosts mood. We will explore different types of exercise and provide guidance on how to incorporate physical activity into your daily routine.

Sleep is often overlooked but is crucial for physical wellbeing. Adequate sleep allows our bodies to rest, recover, and regenerate. We will discuss the importance of establishing a consistent sleep schedule, creating a sleep-friendly environment, and practicing relaxation techniques to promote restful sleep.

Lastly, self-care is an integral part of physical wellbeing. It involves taking time for yourself, engaging in activities that bring you joy and relaxation, and managing stress effectively. We will delve into various self-care practices, including mindfulness, meditation, and stress reduction techniques.

By prioritizing physical wellbeing, we can enhance our overall health and wellbeing. The strategies and tips discussed in this subchapter will empower you to make positive changes in your lifestyle, leading to improved physical health, increased energy levels, and a greater sense of wellbeing. Remember, investing in your physical health is an investment in your happiness and longevity.

Emotional Wellbeing

In today's fast-paced and demanding world, it's crucial to prioritize our emotional wellbeing. Our mental health plays a significant role in our overall wellbeing, affecting our thoughts, feelings, and behaviors. This subchapter aims to shed light on the importance of emotional wellbeing and provide practical strategies to enhance it.

Emotional wellbeing refers to our ability to understand and manage our feelings effectively. It involves recognizing and expressing emotions in a healthy manner, as well as coping with stress, building resilience, and maintaining positive relationships. When we prioritize our emotional wellbeing, we enhance our ability to handle life's challenges and experience greater happiness and fulfillment.

One of the fundamental aspects of emotional wellbeing is self-awareness. It is important to take the time to reflect on our emotions and understand their root causes. By identifying and acknowledging our feelings, we can take steps towards managing them in a healthy and constructive way. This may involve seeking support from loved ones, speaking to a therapist, or engaging in activities that promote relaxation and self-care.

Building emotional resilience is another vital component of emotional wellbeing. Resilience allows us to bounce back from setbacks and adapt to difficult situations. Developing resilience involves nurturing positive thinking patterns, practicing gratitude, and maintaining a growth mindset. By cultivating resilience, we can better navigate the ups and downs of life, reducing the impact of stress on our mental health.

Maintaining healthy relationships is also crucial for emotional wellbeing. Connecting with others and having a support system in place can significantly impact our mental health. It's important to cultivate relationships based on trust, respect, and open communication. By nurturing these connections, we create a sense of belonging and support, which promotes emotional wellbeing.

Additionally, implementing self-care practices is essential for nurturing our emotional wellbeing. Engaging in activities that bring us joy, such as hobbies, exercise, and spending time in nature, can boost our mood and reduce stress. Making time for relaxation, setting healthy boundaries, and practicing mindfulness are also effective strategies to promote emotional wellbeing.

In conclusion, emotional wellbeing is a vital aspect of our overall health and happiness. By prioritizing self-awareness, building resilience, nurturing healthy relationships, and implementing self-care practices, we can enhance our emotional wellbeing. Taking care of our mental health is not only important for ourselves but also for the wellbeing of our communities. By investing in emotional wellbeing, we contribute to the broader public health efforts aimed at creating a society that values and supports mental health for everyone.

Social Wellbeing

Social wellbeing is an essential aspect of our overall mental health and wellbeing. It encompasses the quality of our relationships, our sense of belonging, and our ability to connect and engage with others. In today's fast-paced and digitally-driven world, it is more important than ever to prioritize our social connections and foster a sense of community.

Strong social connections have been proven to have numerous benefits for our mental and physical health. When we have healthy relationships and a sense of belonging, we experience reduced stress levels, improved self-esteem, and a greater sense of purpose and fulfillment. These connections also act as a support system during challenging times, helping us navigate through difficulties and providing emotional and practical assistance.

However, building and maintaining social connections can be challenging, especially in a society that often prioritizes individualism and independence. It requires effort, time, and genuine interest in others. One way to nurture social wellbeing is to actively engage in our communities. This can involve participating in community events, joining clubs or organizations, or volunteering for causes that resonate with us. By doing so, we not only contribute to the greater good but also create opportunities to meet like-minded individuals and form meaningful connections.

Another important aspect of social wellbeing is the quality of our relationships. It is crucial to cultivate healthy and supportive relationships, both with family and friends. This involves open communication, empathy, and mutual respect. It is also important to set boundaries and prioritize self-care to ensure that our relationships are balanced and beneficial to our wellbeing.

In today's digital age, social media has become a significant part of our lives. While it can be a valuable tool for staying connected, it is essential to use it mindfully. Excessive use of social media can lead to feelings of isolation and inadequacy. It is crucial to strike a balance between online and offline interactions and prioritize real-life connections.

In conclusion, social wellbeing is a vital component of mental health and overall wellbeing. By fostering strong social connections, engaging in community activities, and nurturing healthy relationships, we can enhance our social wellbeing. Let us prioritize the quality of our relationships and create a sense of belonging and community in our lives. Together, we can build a society that values social connections and promotes the wellbeing of all individuals.

Spiritual Wellbeing

In our fast-paced and often chaotic world, it is essential to pay attention to not only our physical and mental health but also our spiritual wellbeing. The concept of spiritual wellbeing goes beyond religious beliefs and encompasses a sense of purpose, connection, and inner peace. In this subchapter, we will explore the importance of spiritual wellbeing and how it contributes to our overall mental health and wellbeing.

Spiritual wellbeing is a fundamental aspect of public health, as it plays a significant role in promoting a balanced and fulfilled life. Regardless of one's religious or spiritual beliefs, nurturing our spiritual side can bring about a sense of meaning and purpose, which has been shown to improve our mental and emotional health.

One key aspect of spiritual wellbeing is finding a sense of connection with something greater than ourselves. This can involve developing a connection to nature, engaging in acts of kindness and compassion, or exploring our own personal values and beliefs. By cultivating this connection, we can experience a deeper sense of belonging and find solace during challenging times.

Another essential aspect of spiritual wellbeing is engaging in practices that promote self-reflection and introspection. This can include meditation, prayer, or journaling. These practices enable us to tune in to our inner selves, allowing us to gain insight, clarity, and a deeper understanding of who we are. By engaging in such practices, we can better navigate life's challenges and make decisions that align with our values and aspirations.

Spiritual wellbeing also involves finding a sense of peace and acceptance within ourselves. It encourages us to let go of past grievances, practice forgiveness, and embrace gratitude for the present moment. By cultivating a positive and compassionate mindset, we can experience greater joy and contentment in our lives.

In conclusion, spiritual wellbeing is an integral part of public health and overall wellbeing. Regardless of our religious or spiritual beliefs, nurturing our spiritual side can bring about a sense of purpose, connection, and inner peace. By engaging in practices that promote self-reflection, cultivating a sense of connection, and embracing forgiveness and gratitude, we can enhance our mental and emotional health. Remember, taking care of our spiritual wellbeing is just as important as taking care of our physical and mental health.

Chapter 3: The Mind-Body Connection

Understanding the Mind-Body Connection

In today's fast-paced and stressful world, maintaining good mental health and overall wellbeing is of utmost importance. It is no longer a secret that our minds and bodies are deeply interconnected, and the state of one greatly affects the other. This subchapter aims to shed light on the mind-body connection and its significance in achieving optimal mental health and wellbeing.

The mind-body connection refers to the intricate relationship between our thoughts, emotions, and physical health. It is the realization that our mental state influences our physical health and vice versa. This concept has been acknowledged by ancient healing practices and is now gaining recognition in the field of modern medicine and public health.

Research has shown that stress, anxiety, and negative emotions can have detrimental effects on our physical health. Chronic stress, for example, can lead to a weakened immune system, high blood pressure, and even cardiovascular diseases. Similarly, unresolved emotional trauma can manifest in physical symptoms such as headaches, digestive disorders, or chronic pain.

On the other hand, positive mental states and practices can have a profound impact on our physical wellbeing. Engaging in mindfulness and relaxation techniques, for instance, can reduce stress levels, improve sleep quality, and boost the immune system. Similarly, maintaining a positive mindset and practicing gratitude can enhance overall happiness and satisfaction, leading to a healthier body.

Understanding the mind-body connection empowers individuals to take control of their mental health and make informed decisions to improve their overall wellbeing. It encourages a holistic approach to healthcare, where mental and physical health are treated as interconnected aspects of a person's overall wellness.

In this subchapter, we will delve deeper into the various ways in which the mind and body influence each other. We will explore the impact of stress, emotions, and lifestyle choices on our mental and physical health. Moreover, we will discuss practical strategies and techniques that can help individuals foster a positive mind-body connection and achieve optimal mental health and wellbeing.

By gaining a deeper understanding of the mind-body connection, we can embark on a healing journey that nurtures our mental health and enhances our overall wellbeing. Whether you are a student, a professional, or a parent, this knowledge is invaluable for leading a fulfilling and healthy life. So, let us embark on this transformative journey together and discover the power of the mind-body connection.

Effects of Stress on Mental Health

Stress has become an inevitable part of our lives, affecting individuals from all walks of life. In today's fast-paced world, stressors are often unavoidable, and their impact on mental health cannot be understated. This subchapter aims to shed light on the effects of stress on mental health, providing insights into its implications for individuals' overall wellbeing.

The relationship between stress and mental health is complex and interconnected. Prolonged exposure to stress can have detrimental effects on various aspects of our mental wellbeing. One of the most common consequences of stress is the development or exacerbation of mental health disorders such as anxiety and depression. Stress can act as a catalyst, triggering these conditions or worsening existing symptoms. Furthermore, chronic stress has been linked to an increased risk of developing more severe mental illnesses, such as bipolar disorder or schizophrenia.

Stress also influences cognitive functioning and can impair our ability to concentrate, remember information, and make decisions. It can lead to feelings of overwhelm, affecting our productivity and negatively impacting our professional and personal lives. Additionally, stress can disrupt sleep patterns, leading to insomnia or poor-quality sleep, further exacerbating mental health issues.

Moreover, stress can take a toll on our physical health, indirectly affecting our mental wellbeing. The release of stress hormones, such as cortisol, can weaken our immune system, making us more susceptible to illnesses. The physical symptoms that accompany stress, such as headaches, muscle tension, and gastrointestinal problems, can exacerbate our overall stress levels, creating a vicious cycle between our physical and mental health.

Recognizing the effects of stress on mental health is crucial for public health initiatives. Education and awareness programs can help individuals identify stressors and develop effective coping mechanisms. Encouraging self-care practices, such as exercise, mindfulness, and adequate sleep, can also mitigate the impact of stress on mental wellbeing. Additionally, promoting work-life balance and stress management techniques can empower individuals to prioritize their mental health.

In conclusion, stress has profound effects on mental health, influencing various aspects of our overall wellbeing. Acknowledging the impact of stress is crucial for individuals to take proactive steps towards maintaining their mental health. By addressing stress and implementing strategies to manage it effectively, individuals can enhance their resilience and overall quality of life. In the face of an increasingly stressful world, prioritizing mental health becomes paramount for everyone's wellbeing.

Techniques for Managing Stress

In today's fast-paced world, stress has become an inevitable part of our lives. Whether it is due to work pressures, personal issues, or the ongoing global pandemic, stress can take a toll on our mental and physical health. However, the good news is that there are effective techniques available to manage and reduce stress. By incorporating these techniques into our daily lives, we can improve our overall mental health and wellbeing.

1. Deep Breathing: One of the simplest yet most effective techniques for managing stress is deep breathing. By taking slow, deep breaths and focusing on each inhale and exhale, we can activate the body's relaxation response. Deep breathing helps calm the mind, lowers heart rate, and reduces stress hormones, promoting a sense of calmness and relaxation.

2. Mindfulness Meditation: Mindfulness meditation involves focusing on the present moment without judgment. By practicing mindfulness, we can detach ourselves from stressful thoughts and worries. Regular meditation can help reduce stress, improve concentration, and enhance overall emotional wellbeing.

3. Physical Exercise: Engaging in physical activity has numerous benefits for managing stress. Exercise releases endorphins, the body's natural stress-fighting hormones, which can boost mood and reduce anxiety. Regular exercise also improves sleep quality, increases self-confidence, and provides an outlet for releasing built-up tension.

4. Time Management: Poor time management can lead to increased stress levels. Learning effective time management techniques, such as

prioritizing tasks, setting realistic goals, and scheduling breaks, can help reduce stress and increase productivity. By organizing our time effectively, we can accomplish tasks more efficiently, leaving us with more time for relaxation and self-care.

5. Healthy Lifestyle Choices: Adopting a healthy lifestyle can significantly impact our ability to manage stress. Eating a balanced diet, getting enough sleep, and avoiding excessive caffeine and alcohol consumption can all contribute to better stress management. Additionally, engaging in activities we enjoy, such as hobbies or spending time with loved ones, can provide a much-needed break from stressors.

Remember, managing stress is a continuous process, and what works for one person may not work for another. It's essential to explore and experiment with different techniques to find what suits you best. By incorporating these stress management techniques into our daily routine, we can promote better mental health and overall wellbeing.

In conclusion, stress is a common part of life, but it doesn't have to control us. By practicing deep breathing, mindfulness meditation, engaging in physical exercise, managing our time effectively, and adopting a healthy lifestyle, we can effectively manage and reduce stress levels. Prioritizing our mental health and wellbeing is crucial for leading a fulfilling and balanced life.

The Role of Sleep in Mental Wellbeing

Sleep plays a fundamental role in our overall mental wellbeing. It is a vital component of our daily routine that allows our bodies and minds to rest and rejuvenate. Adequate sleep is essential for maintaining good mental health, and its importance cannot be overstated. In this subchapter, we will delve into the intricate relationship between sleep and mental wellbeing, exploring the various ways that sleep impacts our psychological state.

One of the key functions of sleep is to consolidate our memories and process the information we have gathered throughout the day. During sleep, our brains actively form connections and integrate new knowledge, enhancing our learning and problem-solving abilities. Without sufficient sleep, our cognitive functions become impaired, leading to difficulties in concentration, memory recall, and decision-making.

Furthermore, sleep deprivation has been strongly linked to mental health disorders such as depression and anxiety. Lack of sleep disrupts the delicate balance of chemicals in our brain, specifically serotonin and dopamine, which are crucial for regulating mood and emotions. Consequently, individuals who consistently experience inadequate sleep are more vulnerable to developing mental health conditions and may experience heightened levels of stress, irritability, and emotional instability.

Sleep also plays a significant role in regulating our appetite and metabolism. Sleep deprivation can disrupt the balance of hormones involved in hunger and satiety, leading to increased cravings for unhealthy foods and weight gain. This, in turn, can negatively impact our mental wellbeing by contributing to feelings of low self-esteem and body dissatisfaction.

Additionally, chronic sleep problems can exacerbate existing mental health conditions and hinder the effectiveness of therapeutic interventions. For individuals with conditions such as bipolar disorder or schizophrenia, lack of sleep can trigger manic or psychotic episodes, making it essential to prioritize healthy sleep habits as part of their treatment plan.

To promote mental wellbeing, it is crucial to prioritize sleep hygiene practices. This includes establishing a consistent sleep schedule, creating a comfortable sleep environment, limiting exposure to electronic devices before bedtime, and incorporating relaxation techniques such as meditation or deep breathing exercises. It is also essential to seek professional help if experiencing persistent sleep difficulties or symptoms of mental health disorders.

In conclusion, sleep plays a vital role in maintaining good mental health and overall wellbeing. By understanding the intricate relationship between sleep and mental wellbeing, we can prioritize healthy sleep habits and take the necessary steps to ensure we are getting the restorative sleep we need. By doing so, we can enhance our cognitive functioning, regulate our emotions, and promote optimal mental health for a fulfilling life.

Chapter 4: Nurturing Positive Relationships

The Power of Relationships

In our lives, we often underestimate the profound impact that relationships have on our mental health and overall well-being. Whether it's with family, friends, colleagues, or even strangers, the power of relationships cannot be overlooked. This subchapter aims to shed light on the significant role that relationships play in promoting mental health and well-being, particularly in the context of public health.

Humans are social beings, and our innate need for connection goes beyond mere companionship. Relationships have the power to shape our thoughts, emotions, and behaviors in ways that can either enhance or hinder our mental health. Research has consistently shown that individuals with strong social support networks tend to experience better mental health outcomes, including lower rates of anxiety, depression, and even physical ailments.

One of the primary reasons relationships impact mental health is the emotional support they provide. Having someone to confide in, lean on during challenging times, and share our joys and sorrows with can be immensely therapeutic. Through these connections, we find solace, compassion, and a sense of belonging, all of which are crucial for maintaining good mental health.

Furthermore, relationships also act as a protective factor against various stressors and adversities. In times of crisis, having a support system can help individuals navigate through difficult situations, offering practical assistance, guidance, and a sense of stability. This is particularly relevant in the context of public health, where communities facing health crises or disasters can come together to support one another, mitigating the negative impact on mental health.

Moreover, relationships play a pivotal role in promoting positive health behaviors. When we surround ourselves with individuals who prioritize well-being, we are more likely to adopt and sustain healthy habits ourselves. From encouraging regular exercise to promoting a balanced diet and fostering healthy coping mechanisms, relationships can be a driving force behind positive lifestyle changes.

In the realm of public health, building and nurturing relationships within communities is crucial for creating resilient and supportive environments. By fostering strong social connections, public health initiatives can effectively promote mental health and well-being at a larger scale. This may involve creating platforms for social interaction, organizing community events, or offering support groups that enable individuals to connect with like-minded peers.

In conclusion, the power of relationships cannot be underestimated when it comes to mental health and well-being, especially in the realm of public health. Cultivating strong social connections provides emotional support, acts as a protective factor against stress, and promotes positive health behaviors. By recognizing and harnessing the power of relationships, we can create healthier, happier communities where individuals thrive and support one another on their healing journey towards mental well-being.

Building Healthy Communication

Effective communication is the cornerstone of building healthy relationships, resolving conflicts, and promoting overall wellbeing. In this subchapter, we will explore the various aspects of building healthy communication and how it contributes to mental health and wellbeing. Whether you are a professional in public health or an individual seeking personal growth, mastering the art of communication is crucial for fostering positive connections and creating a healthier society.

First and foremost, healthy communication involves active listening. It is essential to truly hear and understand others, putting aside our own preconceived notions and judgments. When we actively listen, we demonstrate empathy and respect, creating an environment where individuals feel heard and valued. This paves the way for open dialogue and the exchange of ideas, leading to more meaningful and productive conversations.

Another key aspect of healthy communication is effective expression. Being able to clearly and assertively communicate our own thoughts, feelings, and needs is vital for maintaining healthy boundaries and resolving conflicts. By using "I" statements and expressing ourselves in a respectful manner, we can avoid misunderstandings and promote a sense of trust and understanding.

Building healthy communication also involves non-verbal cues. Our body language, facial expressions, and tone of voice play a significant role in how our messages are perceived. Being aware of our non-verbal communication and its impact can help us convey our intentions accurately and build stronger connections with others.

Furthermore, building healthy communication requires cultivating emotional intelligence. Understanding and managing our emotions allows us to respond thoughtfully rather than react impulsively. By practicing empathy, we can better understand the emotions of others and respond in a supportive and compassionate manner.

In the context of public health, healthy communication is essential for disseminating information effectively and promoting behavior change. Clear and concise messaging, tailored to different audiences, can help individuals make informed decisions about their health and wellbeing. It is crucial to use language that is accessible to all, avoiding jargon and taking cultural sensitivities into account.

In conclusion, building healthy communication is a fundamental aspect of promoting mental health and wellbeing. By actively listening, effectively expressing ourselves, being mindful of non-verbal cues, and cultivating emotional intelligence, we can foster positive connections and create a healthier society. Whether you are a public health professional or an individual seeking personal growth, investing in improving your communication skills will undoubtedly contribute to your overall wellbeing and the wellbeing of those around you.

Resolving Conflict

Conflict is an inevitable part of life. It can arise in various aspects of our lives, from our personal relationships to our professional endeavors. Learning how to effectively resolve conflicts is crucial for maintaining our mental health and overall wellbeing. In this subchapter, we will explore strategies and approaches that can help us navigate and resolve conflicts in a healthy and constructive manner.

Understanding the root causes of conflict is the first step towards resolving it. Conflicts often stem from differences in opinions, values, or goals. By acknowledging and respecting these differences, we can create a foundation for open communication and mutual understanding. It is essential to approach conflicts with empathy and a willingness to listen to the perspectives of others, even if they differ from our own.

Communication plays a vital role in conflict resolution. Effective communication involves active listening, expressing oneself clearly and respectfully, and seeking common ground. By actively listening, we can gain insights into the underlying issues and emotions driving the conflict. Expressing ourselves clearly and respectfully allows us to articulate our needs and concerns without attacking or belittling others. Seeking common ground helps us find solutions that accommodate the interests and values of all parties involved.

Managing emotions during conflicts is crucial. Conflicts can trigger strong emotional responses such as anger, frustration, or hurt. Learning how to regulate and express these emotions constructively can prevent conflicts from escalating into harmful or destructive situations. Techniques such as deep breathing, taking breaks, and practicing mindfulness can help us stay calm and focused during tense moments.

Collaboration and compromise are key components of conflict resolution. Instead of approaching conflicts as win-lose situations, we should strive for win-win outcomes where all parties feel their needs and interests are met to some extent. This requires a willingness to find common ground, brainstorm creative solutions, and make necessary compromises. By shifting our mindset from competition to collaboration, we can foster healthier relationships and resolve conflicts more effectively.

In conclusion, conflict resolution is an essential skill for maintaining our mental health and overall wellbeing. By understanding the root causes of conflicts, practicing effective communication, managing emotions, and seeking collaboration and compromise, we can navigate conflicts in a healthy and constructive manner. Resolving conflicts not only strengthens our relationships but also contributes to the overall public health by fostering a more harmonious and peaceful society.

Boundaries in Relationships

In our journey towards mental health and wellbeing, establishing and maintaining healthy boundaries in our relationships plays a crucial role. Boundaries serve as the invisible lines that define where we end and others begin, protecting our physical, emotional, and psychological well-being. They are essential for cultivating healthy and fulfilling relationships.

In the realm of public health, understanding boundaries is of utmost importance. Whether it's our relationships with friends, family members, coworkers, or even strangers, setting boundaries ensures that we maintain our personal space and protect our mental health.

Boundaries allow us to communicate our needs, desires, and limitations effectively. They give us the freedom to say no when necessary and to express our concerns without fear of judgment or rejection. By setting boundaries, we establish a framework that fosters respect, trust, and open communication in our relationships.

Without healthy boundaries, we risk becoming overwhelmed, stressed, and resentful. We may find ourselves constantly sacrificing our own needs for the sake of others, leading to emotional exhaustion and a decline in our overall well-being. By recognizing and setting boundaries, we empower ourselves to prioritize our mental health and establish healthy relationships built on mutual understanding and respect.

Implementing boundaries in our relationships requires self-awareness and assertiveness. It means taking the time to reflect on our own needs and values and communicating them clearly to others. It also involves recognizing when our boundaries are being crossed and taking appropriate action to protect ourselves.

It's important to remember that setting boundaries is not about being selfish or shutting others out. Instead, it's about creating a healthy balance between our own needs and the needs of others. It allows us to show up fully in our relationships, bringing our best selves to the table while honoring our own well-being.

Learning to set and maintain boundaries is a lifelong process that requires practice and self-reflection. It may feel uncomfortable at first, but the rewards are immeasurable. As we establish healthy boundaries, we create a space where both parties can thrive, fostering healthier and more fulfilling relationships.

In conclusion, boundaries in relationships are vital for our mental health and wellbeing. By recognizing and setting boundaries, we protect ourselves from emotional harm and create an environment of respect and understanding. In the realm of public health, understanding and implementing boundaries can lead to healthier communities and stronger relationships. So, let us embark on this healing journey together, prioritizing our mental health and fostering healthy boundaries in all our relationships.

Chapter 5: Developing Self-Awareness

The Importance of Self-Awareness

In the journey towards mental health and overall well-being, one of the most vital aspects is self-awareness. Understanding oneself, our thoughts, emotions, and actions, is an essential foundation for personal growth and maintaining a healthy lifestyle. This subchapter delves into the significance of self-awareness in the context of public health, emphasizing its role in fostering mental health and promoting well-being for everyone.

Self-awareness allows individuals to have a deeper understanding of their own thoughts, feelings, and behaviors. By becoming aware of our emotions and reactions, we can identify patterns and triggers that may be detrimental to our mental health. This knowledge empowers us to make conscious choices and take proactive steps towards positive change. By recognizing our inner struggles, we can seek appropriate support and develop effective coping mechanisms.

Moreover, self-awareness helps us understand the impact of our actions on ourselves and others. In the realm of public health, this awareness is crucial as our behaviors and choices can have far-reaching consequences. By being self-aware, we can make informed decisions that prioritize not only our own well-being but also the health and safety of those around us. This is especially relevant in times of crisis, such as the current global pandemic, where individual actions can significantly impact public health.

Furthermore, self-awareness enables us to recognize and challenge negative self-talk and limiting beliefs. Often, our own internal dialogue can be self-sabotaging and hinder our personal growth. By being aware of these negative patterns, we can reframe our thoughts and cultivate a more positive and constructive mindset. This, in turn, promotes resilience and mental well-being.

In the realm of public health, self-awareness also plays a crucial role in fostering empathy and understanding towards others. By recognizing our own biases, prejudices, and privileges, we can develop a more inclusive and compassionate approach to public health initiatives. This awareness allows us to address disparities and work towards creating equitable and accessible healthcare systems for all.

In conclusion, self-awareness is a fundamental pillar of mental health and overall well-being. By understanding ourselves, our thoughts, emotions, and actions, we can make informed choices, challenge negative patterns, and foster empathy towards others. In the context of public health, self-awareness is vital for promoting individual and collective well-being. It empowers us to prioritize mental health, make responsible decisions, and work towards creating a healthier and more equitable society for everyone.

Exploring Personal Values

In our journey towards mental health and wellbeing, understanding and exploring our personal values is a crucial step. Our values shape our beliefs, behaviors, and decisions, and they play a significant role in our overall happiness and fulfillment. By delving into our values, we gain a deeper understanding of ourselves, our desires, and what truly matters to us. This subchapter aims to guide you through the process of exploring your personal values, helping you uncover the core principles that will lead you towards a healthier and more meaningful life.

Values are the fundamental beliefs that guide our actions and attitudes. They represent what we consider important, and they serve as a compass, directing our behavior and choices. Public health, as a niche, emphasizes the importance of individual values in shaping overall wellbeing and the health of communities.

To begin exploring your personal values, take some time for self-reflection. Ask yourself what principles you hold dear and what qualities you admire in others. Consider the moments when you have felt most fulfilled and content - what values were present in those experiences? Make a list of these values and reflect on how they align with your current lifestyle and goals.

It is also helpful to examine any conflicts between your stated values and your actions. Sometimes, we may unknowingly prioritize certain values over others due to external influences or societal pressures. Identifying these discrepancies allows you to make intentional choices that align with your true values.

Engaging in open and honest conversations with others can further enhance your understanding of values. Discussing your values with loved ones or participating in group activities centered around personal growth and introspection can provide valuable insights and help you gain a broader perspective on what is truly important to you.

Once you have identified your core values, it is important to prioritize them and integrate them into your daily life. By consciously aligning your actions with your values, you will experience a greater sense of authenticity and purpose. Your values will serve as a guiding light, assisting you in making decisions that support your mental health and overall wellbeing.

Exploring personal values is an ongoing process, as our values may evolve and change over time. Regularly revisiting and reassessing your values will ensure that they continue to reflect your true self and guide you towards a life filled with meaning, happiness, and optimal mental health.

Remember, the exploration of personal values is a deeply personal journey, unique to each individual. Embrace this process with an open mind, and allow yourself the space to discover the values that resonate most strongly with you. By doing so, you will embark on a path towards mental health and wellbeing that is authentic and fulfilling.

Identifying Strengths and Weaknesses

In our journey towards mental health and wellbeing, it is crucial to recognize and understand our strengths and weaknesses. This self-awareness is a fundamental step towards personal growth and resilience. By identifying our strengths, we can capitalize on them to build a solid foundation for our mental health. Simultaneously, acknowledging our weaknesses allows us to address and work on them, thereby fostering positive change in our lives.

Strengths are the unique qualities and abilities that define us as individuals. They are the positive attributes that we possess and can draw upon during challenging times. Identifying our strengths helps to boost our self-esteem and confidence, enabling us to navigate life's obstacles with greater resilience. Strengths can manifest in various forms, such as creativity, compassion, determination, or problem-solving skills. By recognizing and appreciating these strengths, we can leverage them to enhance our mental health and overall wellbeing.

On the other hand, weaknesses are areas where we may struggle or face limitations. It is essential to approach weaknesses with compassion and without judgment. Identifying our weaknesses allows us to take an honest inventory of areas in our lives that require improvement or growth. By acknowledging these areas, we can actively seek support, develop coping strategies, or engage in personal development activities to address them. Over time, working on our weaknesses can lead to personal growth and increased mental resilience.

The process of identifying strengths and weaknesses can be facilitated through self-reflection and self-assessment. Taking the time to introspect and explore our thoughts, emotions, and behaviors can provide valuable insights into our strengths and weaknesses. Additionally, seeking feedback from trusted individuals, such as friends, family members, or mentors, can provide an external perspective and help uncover blind spots we may have missed.

Once we have identified our strengths and weaknesses, it is important to remember that they do not define us entirely. We are constantly evolving and capable of growth in all areas of our lives. Embracing our strengths and weaknesses with self-compassion allows us to cultivate a sense of acceptance and understanding. This, in turn, empowers us to make informed decisions, set realistic goals, and take purposeful actions towards our mental health and wellbeing.

In conclusion, identifying strengths and weaknesses is a crucial step in our healing journey towards mental health and wellbeing. By recognizing our strengths, we can leverage them to enhance our resilience and navigate life's challenges. Simultaneously, acknowledging our weaknesses provides an opportunity for growth and personal development. Embracing both aspects with self-compassion and a growth mindset allows us to embark on a path of self-discovery and transformation.

Practicing Self-Compassion

In the pursuit of mental health and wellbeing, one often overlooks the importance of self-compassion. We tend to be our own harshest critics, constantly judging ourselves and setting impossibly high standards. However, cultivating self-compassion is crucial for our overall wellbeing and can significantly impact our mental health.

Self-compassion can be defined as extending the same kindness, care, and understanding to ourselves that we would offer to a loved one. It involves acknowledging our own suffering and treating ourselves with kindness and empathy. This practice allows us to respond to our own pain and challenges with understanding and gentleness, fostering a sense of self-worth and resilience.

In today's fast-paced and demanding world, it is crucial that we prioritize self-compassion. Public health research has shown that individuals who practice self-compassion experience lower levels of stress, anxiety, and depression. They also have higher levels of life satisfaction, resilience, and overall wellbeing.

When we practice self-compassion, we learn to embrace our imperfections and treat ourselves with kindness. Instead of engaging in negative self-talk or self-criticism, we cultivate a mindset of self-acceptance and self-love. We recognize that making mistakes and facing challenges are part of the human experience, and we respond to ourselves with understanding and support.

Developing self-compassion requires practice and patience. It involves being mindful of our own thoughts and emotions and challenging negative self-judgments. We can start by reframing our inner dialogue, replacing self-criticism with self-encouragement. We can remind ourselves that we are doing the best we can and that it is okay to make mistakes.

Engaging in self-care activities is also an important aspect of self-compassion. Taking time for ourselves, engaging in activities that bring us joy and relaxation, and prioritizing our physical and emotional needs are all ways to practice self-compassion. By nurturing ourselves, we fill our own cup and become better equipped to navigate the challenges that life throws at us.

In conclusion, self-compassion is an essential component of mental health and wellbeing. By treating ourselves with kindness, understanding, and care, we can cultivate a sense of self-worth and resilience. Practicing self-compassion allows us to embrace our imperfections and respond to our own pain and challenges with love and empathy. So, let us make a conscious effort to prioritize self-compassion in our lives and experience the transformative power it has to offer.

Chapter 6: Cultivating Resilience

Understanding Resilience

Resilience is a fundamental aspect of mental health and wellbeing that allows individuals to adapt, bounce back, and thrive in the face of adversity. In the context of public health, understanding resilience becomes crucial as it enables us to develop effective strategies and interventions to support individuals and communities in their healing journey.

Resilience is not a fixed trait or something that only a few lucky individuals possess. It is a skill that can be cultivated and strengthened over time. It involves developing coping mechanisms, problem-solving abilities, and emotional regulation techniques that help individuals navigate difficult situations and emerge stronger.

One important aspect of understanding resilience is recognizing that it is not about avoiding stress or challenges altogether. Rather, it is about building the capacity to effectively manage and overcome them. Resilient individuals possess a positive outlook, a sense of purpose, and the ability to adapt to changing circumstances.

Resilience is a multidimensional concept that encompasses various factors, including social support, self-esteem, and optimism. Having a strong support network, whether it be family, friends, or community, plays a vital role in bolstering resilience. Connecting with others, seeking help when needed, and fostering positive relationships can significantly enhance an individual's ability to cope with adversity.

Self-esteem and self-confidence are also integral to resilience. By cultivating a positive self-image and believing in one's abilities, individuals are better equipped to face challenges head-on. Furthermore, optimism and a growth mindset enable individuals to view setbacks as opportunities for growth and learning, rather than insurmountable obstacles.

Understanding resilience also involves acknowledging the impact of adverse childhood experiences (ACEs) on mental health and wellbeing. ACEs, such as abuse, neglect, or household dysfunction, can have long-lasting effects on individuals' resilience. However, by providing trauma-informed care and support, we can help individuals overcome the lasting effects of ACEs and build resilience.

In conclusion, understanding resilience is essential for promoting mental health and wellbeing within the realm of public health. It involves recognizing resilience as a skill that can be developed and strengthened through various factors such as social support, self-esteem, and optimism. By fostering resilience in individuals and communities, we can empower them to navigate life's challenges and thrive in the face of adversity.

Strategies for Building Resilience

In today's fast-paced and ever-changing world, it is essential to cultivate resilience to maintain mental health and overall well-being. Resilience refers to the ability to bounce back from adversity, cope with stress, and adapt to challenging situations. It is a skill that can be developed and strengthened through various strategies. This subchapter explores some effective strategies for building resilience that can benefit everyone, with a particular focus on the field of public health.

First and foremost, developing a strong support network is vital for building resilience. Surrounding yourself with positive and supportive individuals can provide emotional support, encouragement, and guidance during difficult times. Engaging in regular social interactions, participating in community activities, and maintaining healthy relationships are all ways to foster a robust support system.

Another strategy for building resilience is developing healthy coping mechanisms. This involves identifying and implementing healthy ways to manage stress and emotions. Some effective coping strategies include engaging in physical exercise, practicing mindfulness and meditation, cultivating hobbies and interests, and seeking professional help when needed. These strategies not only help individuals cope with stress but also enhance their overall mental well-being.

Building resilience also requires embracing change and developing a growth mindset. Accepting that change is a natural part of life and focusing on personal growth can help individuals navigate through challenging circumstances. This mindset enables individuals to view setbacks as opportunities for learning and personal development rather than as failures.

Furthermore, self-care plays a vital role in building resilience. Taking care of one's physical, emotional, and mental health is crucial for overall well-being. Engaging in activities that promote self-care, such as getting enough sleep, eating a balanced diet, practicing relaxation techniques, and engaging in enjoyable activities, can significantly contribute to building resilience.

Lastly, maintaining a positive outlook and practicing gratitude are key components of resilience. Cultivating optimism and gratitude can help individuals reframe negative experiences and find meaning and purpose in life's challenges. Expressing gratitude for the positive aspects of life can enhance overall well-being and resilience.

In conclusion, building resilience is essential for maintaining mental health and well-being in today's fast-paced world. By developing a strong support network, adopting healthy coping mechanisms, embracing change and growth, practicing self-care, and maintaining a positive outlook, individuals can cultivate resilience and thrive in the face of adversity. These strategies are particularly relevant in the field of public health, where resilience is crucial for addressing the challenges that arise in promoting the well-being of communities and populations.

Overcoming Adversity

Life is full of ups and downs, and at some point, we all face adversity. It is during these challenging times that our mental health and wellbeing can be put to the test. In this subchapter, we will explore the concept of overcoming adversity and provide practical strategies to help you navigate through difficult times.

Adversity comes in many forms – it could be a personal loss, a health issue, financial struggles, or even a global crisis. Regardless of the nature of the challenge, it is important to remember that you are not alone. Adversity is a universal experience, and countless individuals have successfully overcome similar obstacles before you. By understanding this, you can draw strength from the collective resilience of humanity.

One of the first steps in overcoming adversity is acknowledging and accepting your emotions. It is absolutely normal to feel sadness, anger, fear, or frustration during tough times. Give yourself permission to experience and express these emotions in a healthy way. This could involve talking to a trusted friend or family member, journaling, or seeking professional help if needed.

Developing a positive mindset is crucial in overcoming adversity. Instead of dwelling on the negative aspects of the situation, try to focus on the lessons and opportunities for growth. This shift in perspective can help you find meaning and purpose in the face of adversity.

Another important aspect of overcoming adversity is building a support network. Surround yourself with people who uplift and inspire you. Lean on your loved ones for emotional support, seek guidance from mentors or counselors, and consider joining support groups where you can connect with others who have faced similar challenges. Remember, seeking help is a sign of strength, not weakness.

Taking care of your physical and mental wellbeing is essential during difficult times. Engage in activities that bring you joy and relaxation, such as exercise, meditation, or pursuing hobbies. Practice self-care and prioritize self-compassion. Be patient with yourself and allow yourself time to heal and recover.

Overcoming adversity is not an overnight process. It requires resilience, determination, and a willingness to face your fears head-on. Remember that setbacks are a part of the journey, and it is through these setbacks that we learn and grow. Embrace the challenges, believe in your ability to overcome, and trust that you have the strength within you to triumph over any adversity.

In conclusion, overcoming adversity is a universal experience that requires resilience and a positive mindset. By acknowledging your emotions, building a support network, and taking care of your wellbeing, you can navigate through difficult times and emerge stronger than ever before. Remember, you are not alone, and with the right tools and mindset, you can overcome any adversity that life throws your way.

Embracing Change

Embracing Change: Navigating the Path to Mental Health and Wellbeing

Change is an inevitable part of life, and learning to embrace it is crucial for our mental health and overall wellbeing. In this subchapter, we will explore the transformative power of embracing change and how it can positively impact our lives.

Change can be both exciting and intimidating, but it is through change that we grow and evolve as individuals. In the realm of public health, embracing change is essential for addressing and improving societal well-being. Whether it is adapting to new technologies, implementing innovative healthcare systems, or promoting mental health awareness, change is the driving force behind progress.

One of the first steps towards embracing change is cultivating a mindset of openness and flexibility. By being receptive to new ideas and perspectives, we allow ourselves to see opportunities where others may only see obstacles. Public health professionals, in particular, must be willing to adapt and modify strategies to meet the evolving needs of communities.

Embracing change also involves letting go of fear and resistance. Change often brings uncertainty, and it is natural to feel apprehensive about the unknown. However, by acknowledging our fears and challenging them, we can discover new possibilities and personal growth. This is especially relevant in the field of public health, where professionals must confront complex challenges and advocate for necessary changes in policy and practice.

Additionally, embracing change requires resilience and a willingness to learn from our experiences. It is essential to view setbacks as opportunities for growth and to remain open to feedback and self-reflection. By embracing change, we can adapt to new circumstances, acquire new skills, and foster personal and professional development.

In the context of public health, embracing change involves recognizing the dynamic nature of our society and the need for continuous improvement. It requires a commitment to staying informed about emerging research, new technologies, and innovative approaches. By embracing change, public health professionals can drive positive transformations in healthcare systems, policies, and public attitudes towards mental health.

Ultimately, embracing change is a powerful catalyst for personal and societal transformation. When we embrace change, we open ourselves up to new possibilities, expand our horizons, and foster resilience. In the context of public health, embracing change is crucial for addressing the evolving needs of communities and promoting mental health and wellbeing for all.

In summary, this subchapter on "Embracing Change" highlights the importance of adopting a positive mindset, overcoming fear and resistance, and remaining resilient in the face of change. It emphasizes the significance of embracing change in public health, where it serves as a driving force for progress and improved wellbeing. By embracing change, we can navigate the path towards mental health and overall wellbeing, both individually and as a society.

Chapter 7: Seeking Help and Support

Recognizing When to Seek Help

In our journey towards mental health and wellbeing, it is crucial to recognize when seeking help is necessary. Mental health issues can affect anyone, regardless of age, gender, or background. Unfortunately, many individuals struggle in silence, unaware that support and assistance are readily available.

Recognizing the signs that indicate the need for professional help is vital. Some common indicators include persistent feelings of sadness, hopelessness, or anxiety that interfere with daily functioning. Other warning signs may include changes in appetite or sleep patterns, loss of interest in activities once enjoyed, difficulty concentrating, or thoughts of self-harm or suicide.

One of the first steps in recognizing the need for help is acknowledging that mental health is just as important as physical health. Just as we would seek medical attention for a physical ailment, it is crucial to approach our mental health with the same care and concern.

Public health initiatives play a significant role in raising awareness about mental health and encouraging individuals to seek help. By providing education and disseminating information, public health campaigns can help reduce the stigma surrounding mental health issues, making it easier for people to reach out for assistance.

It is important to remember that seeking help is not a sign of weakness but a brave and necessary step towards healing. Mental health professionals, such as psychologists, psychiatrists, and therapists, are trained to provide support, guidance, and evidence-based treatments to individuals experiencing mental health challenges.

When considering seeking help, it is essential to reach out to a trusted professional or a helpline specifically designed to provide mental health support. These professionals can assist in assessing the severity of the situation and recommend appropriate interventions. They can also provide information about local resources and support networks that can aid in the healing process.

Remember, you are not alone in your struggles. Many individuals have faced similar challenges and found solace and support through seeking help. By recognizing when to seek assistance and taking that crucial step, you are prioritizing your mental health and taking an active role in your own wellbeing.

In conclusion, recognizing when to seek help is a vital aspect of our healing journey towards mental health and wellbeing. By acknowledging the signs and symptoms of mental health issues, understanding the importance of mental health, and seeking assistance from professionals, we can ensure that we receive the support and care we need. Remember, there is no shame in reaching out for help - it is a courageous act that can lead to a brighter, healthier future.

Types of Mental Health Professionals

In the field of mental health, there are many professionals who play a vital role in promoting and maintaining our psychological well-being. These professionals possess the necessary knowledge and expertise to help individuals cope with life's challenges, navigate through difficult emotions, and achieve optimal mental health. This subchapter explores the different types of mental health professionals and the unique contributions they make in the field.

1. Psychiatrists: Psychiatrists are medical doctors who specialize in mental health. They can diagnose and treat mental illnesses, prescribe medication, and provide therapy. These professionals often work with individuals who have severe mental health conditions such as schizophrenia, bipolar disorder, or major depressive disorder.

2. Psychologists: Psychologists are experts in the field of human behavior and mental processes. They hold advanced degrees in psychology and are trained in various therapeutic techniques. Psychologists can provide counseling and therapy for individuals with a wide range of mental health concerns, such as anxiety, phobias, or relationship issues.

3. Counselors: Counselors, also known as mental health counselors or therapists, work with individuals, families, and groups to address emotional and mental health challenges. They provide support, guidance, and therapeutic interventions to help individuals improve their overall well-being. Counselors often specialize in specific areas such as addiction, grief, or trauma.

4. Social Workers: Social workers are trained professionals who help individuals and families overcome social and emotional difficulties. They provide counseling, advocacy, and connect individuals with community resources. Social workers may work in various settings, such as hospitals, schools, or community organizations, to address a wide range of mental health concerns.

5. Psychiatric Nurses: Psychiatric nurses are registered nurses who specialize in mental health. They work closely with psychiatrists and other mental health professionals to provide comprehensive care to individuals with mental illnesses. Psychiatric nurses may administer medication, provide counseling, and educate patients and their families about managing their mental health conditions.

6. Peer Support Specialists: Peer support specialists are individuals who have personal experience with mental health challenges and are trained to provide support to others facing similar circumstances. They offer empathy, understanding, and guidance based on their own recovery journey. Peer support can be invaluable in helping individuals feel understood and supported.

7. Occupational Therapists: Occupational therapists focus on helping individuals develop the skills necessary to engage in meaningful activities and improve their overall well-being. They work with individuals with mental health conditions to develop coping strategies, enhance daily functioning, and improve quality of life.

It is essential to recognize that mental health professionals work collaboratively, often in interdisciplinary teams, to provide comprehensive care. The combination of their expertise and knowledge ensures that individuals receive the most appropriate and effective interventions for their mental health concerns.

Understanding the roles and contributions of different mental health professionals can empower individuals to seek appropriate support and make informed decisions about their mental health care. Whether you are seeking therapy, medication management, or ongoing support, there is a mental health professional available to help you on your healing journey towards mental health and wellbeing.

Therapy Options

When it comes to addressing mental health and wellbeing, therapy is an essential tool that can help individuals navigate their healing journey. Therapy options are diverse and tailored to meet the specific needs and preferences of each individual. Whether you are struggling with anxiety, depression, trauma, or any other mental health concern, therapy can provide you with the support and guidance you need to overcome these challenges.

One commonly known therapy option is psychotherapy, also referred to as talk therapy. This approach involves discussing your thoughts, feelings, and experiences with a trained therapist. Psychotherapy can help you gain insight into your emotions, develop coping mechanisms, and work towards resolving past traumas. Cognitive-behavioral therapy (CBT) is a specific type of psychotherapy that focuses on identifying and challenging negative thought patterns and behaviors, promoting healthier ways of thinking and behaving.

Another therapy option is medication management. In some cases, mental health conditions may be alleviated or managed with the help of medication prescribed by a psychiatrist. Medication can balance brain chemicals and reduce symptoms associated with mental health disorders. However, it is important to note that medication alone is not a comprehensive solution, and it is often combined with therapy for optimal results.

For individuals who prefer alternative approaches, there are various holistic therapy options available. These include art therapy, music therapy, mindfulness-based therapy, and animal-assisted therapy.

These therapies recognize the interconnectedness of the mind, body, and spirit and aim to promote healing through creative expression, relaxation techniques, and the companionship of animals.

In recent years, technology has also revolutionized therapy options. Online therapy, also known as teletherapy or e-therapy, allows individuals to receive therapy from the comfort of their own homes through video calls or messaging platforms. Online therapy has made mental health support more accessible and convenient for many people, particularly those with limited mobility or in remote areas.

It is important to remember that therapy options are not one-size-fits-all. What works for one person may not work for another. It may take some trial and error to find the therapy option that resonates with you and your unique circumstances. However, the most significant step is recognizing that seeking therapy is a courageous and empowering choice on your healing journey.

By exploring therapy options, you are taking an active role in improving your mental health and wellbeing. Remember, you are not alone in this journey, and there is help available for everyone. Don't hesitate to reach out to a mental health professional to discuss the therapy options that could best support your needs and lead you towards a path of healing and wellbeing.

Support Networks and Resources

In our journey towards mental health and wellbeing, it is crucial to recognize the significance of support networks and resources available to us. These invaluable tools can provide the necessary guidance, assistance, and encouragement when navigating the ups and downs of life. Regardless of who we are or where we come from, support networks and resources play a vital role in promoting our mental health and overall wellbeing.

Support networks are the individuals, groups, and communities that surround us and offer their understanding, empathy, and assistance. They can include family, friends, colleagues, mentors, and even online communities. These networks provide a sense of belonging, validation, and emotional support during challenging times. Whether we are facing a mental health crisis or simply need someone to talk to, support networks are there to lend a listening ear and offer a helping hand.

However, it is important to remember that support networks are not limited to our immediate circles. There are numerous resources available within the realm of public health that can significantly contribute to our mental health journey. These resources encompass a wide spectrum of services and organizations dedicated to promoting mental wellbeing and providing assistance when needed.

One such resource is mental health hotlines, which are available 24/7 and offer confidential support and guidance to individuals in crisis. These hotlines are staffed by trained professionals who can provide immediate intervention, listen to concerns, and offer resources for further support.

Support groups are another valuable resource within the public health sphere. These groups bring together individuals facing similar challenges, such as addiction, grief, or anxiety, and provide a safe space to share experiences, gain insights, and receive encouragement. Support groups foster a sense of community and offer a platform for individuals to learn from one another's journeys.

Public health initiatives and organizations also play a crucial role in promoting mental health and wellbeing. These initiatives focus on raising awareness, reducing stigma, and providing education about mental health. They often offer workshops, seminars, and online resources to empower individuals with knowledge and skills to manage their mental health effectively.

In conclusion, support networks and resources are essential components of our healing journey towards mental health and wellbeing. They provide us with the necessary tools, guidance, and understanding to navigate life's challenges successfully. Whether it be through our personal support networks or the resources available within public health, we can find solace, strength, and encouragement in knowing that we are not alone on this path. Let us embrace the support networks and resources available to us, allowing them to guide us towards a life of improved mental health and overall wellbeing.

Chapter 8: Lifestyle Factors for Mental Wellbeing

Diet and Nutrition

In the pursuit of mental health and overall well-being, diet and nutrition play a crucial role that should not be overlooked. The food we consume not only fuels our bodies but also affects our mental and emotional states. This subchapter will explore the significant impact of diet and nutrition on mental health, providing valuable insights and practical tips for everyone interested in enhancing their well-being.

A balanced diet that includes a variety of nutrients is essential for maintaining optimal mental health. Nutrient deficiencies can lead to various mental health issues, such as depression, anxiety, and even cognitive decline. Therefore, it is important to ensure that our daily diet consists of a wide range of fruits, vegetables, whole grains, lean proteins, and healthy fats.

One nutrient that has gained significant attention in recent years is omega-3 fatty acids. These essential fats are found in abundance in oily fish, nuts, and seeds. Research suggests that omega-3 fatty acids have a positive impact on mood regulation and can potentially reduce the risk of depression and anxiety. Incorporating sources of omega-3s into our diet can be beneficial for our mental well-being.

Additionally, the gut-brain connection has emerged as a fascinating area of research in recent years. The gut microbiota, the millions of bacteria residing in our digestive system, have been found to influence our mental health. A healthy gut microbiome, supported by a diet rich in fiber, prebiotics, and probiotics, can contribute to better mental health outcomes. Fermented foods like yogurt, sauerkraut, and kefir are excellent sources of probiotics that promote a healthy gut.

It is important to note that individual nutritional needs may vary, and it is always recommended to consult with a healthcare professional or registered dietitian for personalized guidance. They can provide tailored advice based on specific health conditions, dietary restrictions, and personal goals.

In conclusion, diet and nutrition are vital components of our mental health and overall well-being. By adopting a well-balanced diet that includes essential nutrients, such as omega-3 fatty acids, and prioritizing gut health through the consumption of probiotics and fiber-rich foods, we can support our mental well-being. Remember, small changes in our diet can lead to significant improvements in our mental health, making it an essential aspect of our healing journey towards greater mental health and well-being.

Regular Exercise and Physical Activity

In today's fast-paced world, it is becoming increasingly important to prioritize our physical health and wellbeing. Regular exercise and physical activity play a vital role in maintaining good overall health and preventing a range of chronic diseases. This subchapter aims to shed light on the importance of incorporating regular exercise into our daily lives, and how it can contribute to our mental health and wellbeing.

Physical activity is not just about hitting the gym or participating in organized sports; it encompasses any bodily movement that requires energy expenditure. Engaging in regular physical activity has numerous benefits for everyone, regardless of age, gender, or fitness level. From reducing the risk of heart disease and stroke to improving bone and muscle strength, physical activity is a key component of public health.

Regular exercise not only improves our physical health but also has a significant impact on our mental wellbeing. Research has shown that physical activity can help reduce symptoms of depression and anxiety, boost mood, and improve overall cognitive function. Engaging in exercise releases endorphins, also known as "feel-good" hormones, which can contribute to a sense of happiness and relaxation.

Furthermore, regular exercise can enhance our sleep quality, increase our energy levels, and improve our self-esteem. It provides an opportunity to disconnect from the stresses of daily life and focus on taking care of ourselves. Incorporating physical activity into our routine can also promote social interaction and strengthen our relationships, whether through joining group classes or participating in team sports.

It is important to note that physical activity does not have to be excessive or strenuous to reap the benefits. Even moderate-intensity activities, such as brisk walking, swimming, or gardening, can have a positive impact on our health and wellbeing. The key is to find activities that we enjoy and can realistically incorporate into our daily lives.

In conclusion, regular exercise and physical activity are essential for maintaining good overall health and promoting mental wellbeing. Whether it's through cardiovascular exercises, strength training, or simply staying active throughout the day, the benefits are abundant. By prioritizing physical activity, we can improve our physical health, boost our mood, reduce stress, and enhance our overall quality of life. So, let's take the first step towards a healthier and happier future by incorporating regular exercise into our daily routines.

Mindfulness and Meditation

Mindfulness and Meditation: Cultivating Mental Health and Wellbeing

In today's fast-paced and chaotic world, it's easy to become overwhelmed by the demands and stresses of everyday life. Public health concerns are on the rise, as people struggle to find effective ways to cope with the pressures that impact their mental health and overall wellbeing. This subchapter on mindfulness and meditation aims to provide a comprehensive understanding of these practices and their role in promoting mental health for everyone.

Mindfulness is the practice of paying attention to the present moment, with an open and non-judgmental attitude. By bringing awareness to our thoughts, feelings, and bodily sensations, we can develop a deeper understanding of ourselves and the world around us. This heightened awareness allows us to respond to life's challenges with greater clarity and compassion, improving our mental and emotional resilience.

Meditation, on the other hand, is a deliberate and focused technique that aims to calm the mind and promote relaxation. By engaging in various meditation practices, such as breathing exercises or guided imagery, individuals can achieve a state of deep relaxation, reducing stress and anxiety. Regular meditation has been shown to have a myriad of positive effects on mental health, including improved concentration, emotional stability, and overall happiness.

Research has shown that mindfulness and meditation can have a profound impact on public health. They have been proven effective in reducing symptoms of depression, anxiety, and stress-related disorders. Moreover, mindfulness-based interventions have shown promising results in managing chronic pain, boosting the immune system, and even enhancing cognitive functions.

This subchapter will delve into the science behind mindfulness and meditation, exploring the neurological and physiological mechanisms that underlie their benefits. It will also provide practical guidance on how to incorporate these practices into our daily lives, even amidst our busy schedules. From simple breathing exercises to guided meditation sessions, the tools and techniques shared here will empower readers to embark on their own healing journey towards mental health and wellbeing.

Whether you are a student, a working professional, or a retiree, this subchapter will offer valuable insights and strategies for cultivating mindfulness and meditation in your life. By adopting these practices, we can enhance our mental health, reduce stress, and promote overall wellbeing, contributing to a healthier and happier society at large. Let us embark on this journey together towards a more mindful and compassionate world.

Hobbies and Leisure Activities

In our fast-paced and demanding lives, it is crucial to prioritize our mental health and wellbeing. While many factors contribute to our overall mental state, including professional success, personal relationships, and physical health, one often overlooked aspect is our leisure time. Engaging in hobbies and leisure activities can be a powerful tool for improving mental health and promoting overall wellbeing.

Hobbies and leisure activities offer a much-needed break from the daily stresses and pressures of life. They provide an opportunity to disconnect from work and responsibilities and indulge in activities that bring us joy and fulfillment. Whether it's painting, gardening, playing a musical instrument, or even just taking a leisurely walk in nature, these activities allow us to recharge and rejuvenate.

Engaging in hobbies and leisure activities can also serve as a form of self-care. By dedicating time to activities we love, we prioritize our own needs and promote self-compassion. This can have a profound impact on our mental health, as it helps us develop a positive relationship with ourselves and cultivate a sense of self-worth.

Furthermore, hobbies and leisure activities have been shown to reduce stress and anxiety. When we immerse ourselves in activities we enjoy, our minds shift focus, and our stress levels decrease. Engaging in these activities also promotes the release of endorphins, the body's natural feel-good chemicals, which can boost our mood and overall sense of wellbeing.

For individuals in the field of public health, promoting hobbies and leisure activities can have significant implications for the overall wellbeing of communities. Encouraging individuals to engage in activities they enjoy can improve mental health outcomes, reduce stress-related illnesses, and enhance overall quality of life. Public health professionals can play a vital role in providing resources, organizing community events, and advocating for the integration of leisure activities into everyday life.

In conclusion, hobbies and leisure activities are not just mere pastimes; they are essential for our mental health and wellbeing. By setting aside time for activities we enjoy, we can recharge, reduce stress, and promote self-care. For public health professionals, recognizing the importance of hobbies and leisure activities can lead to improved community mental health outcomes. So, let us all prioritize our hobbies and leisure activities, and embark on a healing journey towards enhanced mental health and wellbeing.

Chapter 9: Promoting Mental Health in the Workplace

The Importance of Mental Health at Work

In today's fast-paced and competitive world, the significance of mental health at work cannot be overstated. As we spend a significant portion of our lives in the workplace, it is crucial to prioritize our mental well-being in this setting. This subchapter aims to shed light on the importance of mental health at work and its impact on both individuals and organizations.

Mental health refers to our emotional, psychological, and social well-being. It affects how we think, feel, and act, and influences how we handle stress, relate to others, and make choices. With work-related stress becoming increasingly prevalent, it is essential to understand the impact it has on our mental health.

For individuals, maintaining good mental health at work is crucial for overall well-being. It enables us to perform at our best, make informed decisions, and handle challenges effectively. A positive mental state promotes creativity, productivity, and job satisfaction. Conversely, poor mental health can lead to decreased concentration, reduced productivity, and increased absenteeism. It can also contribute to the development of mental illnesses such as anxiety and depression.

From an organizational perspective, investing in mental health initiatives is beneficial for both employees and the company as a whole. By creating a supportive and inclusive work environment, organizations can promote employee engagement and loyalty. When employees feel valued and supported, they are more likely to be motivated, productive, and committed to their work. Additionally, prioritizing mental health can lead to reduced healthcare costs and decreased turnover rates, ultimately improving the bottom line.

Public health plays a crucial role in promoting mental health at work. By advocating for policies that prioritize mental health, public health professionals can contribute to the creation of mentally healthy workplaces. This includes implementing strategies to reduce work-related stress, providing access to mental health resources, and promoting a culture that values well-being.

In conclusion, the importance of mental health at work cannot be underestimated. It directly impacts individuals' well-being and plays a significant role in organizational success. Prioritizing mental health in the workplace can lead to improved productivity, increased job satisfaction, and reduced healthcare costs. Public health professionals have a crucial role to play in advocating for mental health initiatives and creating mentally healthy workplaces. By recognizing the importance of mental health at work, we can embark on a healing journey towards discovering mental health and well-being for everyone.

Creating a Supportive Work Environment

In today's fast-paced and demanding world, it is crucial to prioritize mental health and wellbeing, especially in the workplace. A supportive work environment plays a pivotal role in promoting overall wellness and preventing mental health issues. This subchapter aims to guide individuals and organizations in public health towards creating a nurturing and empowering work environment for everyone.

First and foremost, fostering open communication is essential. Encouraging employees to express their thoughts, concerns, and ideas without fear of judgment or retribution is vital. Regular team meetings, one-on-one sessions, and suggestion boxes can provide platforms for individuals to voice their opinions. By actively listening and valuing their input, organizations can cultivate a culture of trust and collaboration.

Another crucial aspect is promoting work-life balance. In today's hyperconnected world, it is increasingly difficult to separate personal and professional lives. Encouraging employees to set boundaries and prioritize self-care can significantly improve their overall mental wellbeing. Flexible work hours, remote work options, and wellness programs can help individuals achieve a healthy balance between work and personal life.

Building a supportive work environment also involves providing opportunities for growth and development. Offering training programs, workshops, and mentorship initiatives can enhance employees' skills and boost their confidence. Recognizing and rewarding achievements further motivates individuals to strive for excellence.

Additionally, promoting a positive work culture and fostering strong relationships among colleagues is crucial. Encouraging teamwork, empathy, and respect creates a sense of belonging and camaraderie within the workplace. Celebrating milestones, organizing team-building activities, and promoting diversity and inclusion can further strengthen the bond between team members.

Lastly, it is important to address and destigmatize mental health issues. Incorporating mental health awareness programs, providing access to counseling services, and educating employees about available resources can help individuals seek help when needed. Organizations should also implement policies that prioritize mental health, such as offering mental health days or flexible sick leave policies.

Creating a supportive work environment is an ongoing process that requires commitment and dedication. By prioritizing mental health and wellbeing, organizations in public health can foster a culture that not only benefits employees but also enhances productivity and overall organizational success. Together, let us strive towards creating workplaces where mental health is valued, and every individual can thrive.

Reducing Work-Related Stress

In today's fast-paced and demanding world, work-related stress has become a significant concern for individuals across all walks of life. Whether you are a corporate executive, a healthcare professional, or a teacher, the pressures of the workplace can take a toll on your mental health and overall wellbeing. This subchapter aims to provide valuable insights and practical strategies to help individuals effectively manage and reduce work-related stress.

Recognizing the signs of work-related stress is the first step towards addressing this issue. Often, we may not even realize that we are experiencing stress until it begins to manifest physically or emotionally. Symptoms such as fatigue, irritability, difficulty concentrating, and even physical ailments like headaches or stomachaches can all be indicators of work-related stress. By becoming more aware of these signs, individuals can take proactive measures to alleviate stress before it becomes overwhelming.

One effective strategy for reducing work-related stress is to establish clear boundaries between work and personal life. In today's digital age, it is easy to be constantly connected to work through smartphones and laptops, blurring the line between professional and personal time. Setting specific time limits for work-related activities, such as checking emails or taking work calls, can help create a healthier work-life balance and reduce the risk of burnout.

Another important aspect of reducing work-related stress is fostering a supportive and positive work environment. Employers and managers play a crucial role in creating an atmosphere that promotes mental health and wellbeing. Encouraging open communication, providing resources for stress management, and implementing flexible work arrangements can all contribute to a healthier workplace culture.

Additionally, self-care practices can greatly aid in reducing work-related stress. Engaging in activities that promote relaxation and rejuvenation, such as exercise, meditation, or hobbies, can help individuals recharge and manage stress effectively. Prioritizing self-care may require individuals to carve out dedicated time for themselves, but the long-term benefits are worth it.

Finally, seeking professional help should not be overlooked. If work-related stress becomes overwhelming and begins to impact one's mental health, it is crucial to consult with a mental health professional who can provide guidance and support. Therapy or counseling can equip individuals with coping mechanisms and strategies to navigate work-related stress more effectively.

In conclusion, work-related stress is a pressing issue that affects individuals from all walks of life. By recognizing the signs of stress, establishing boundaries, fostering a supportive work environment, practicing self-care, and seeking professional help when needed, individuals can effectively reduce work-related stress and pave the way for improved mental health and overall wellbeing.

Employee Assistance Programs

Employee Assistance Programs (EAPs) play a vital role in promoting mental health and wellbeing in the workplace. In today's fast-paced and demanding world, it is crucial for employers to provide resources and support systems that address the mental health needs of their employees. This subchapter explores the concept of Employee Assistance Programs and their significance in public health.

Employee Assistance Programs are employer-sponsored initiatives designed to assist employees in managing personal and work-related challenges that may impact their mental health. These programs provide a range of services, including counseling, education, referral services, and wellness initiatives. The primary goal is to create a supportive environment that enables employees to cope with stress, enhance productivity, and achieve a work-life balance.

In recent years, the importance of EAPs has gained recognition due to the growing awareness of mental health issues in the workplace. Stress, anxiety, depression, and burnout have become prevalent, affecting employees' overall wellbeing and productivity. EAPs offer a proactive approach to addressing these challenges, allowing employees to seek assistance before their mental health deteriorates.

The benefits of EAPs extend beyond individual employees to the organization as a whole. By investing in the mental health and wellbeing of their workforce, employers can reduce absenteeism, turnover rates, and healthcare costs. They also contribute to creating a positive work culture that values employee wellbeing and fosters a sense of belonging.

Public health experts widely recommend the integration of EAPs into workplace policies and practices. These programs promote mental health awareness, reduce stigma, and provide a safe space for employees to seek support. By acknowledging and addressing mental health concerns, organizations contribute to the overall improvement of public health.

EAPs are not limited to large corporations; they can be implemented by organizations of all sizes. Employers can customize these programs to meet the specific needs and resources of their workforce. Whether it is through offering counseling sessions, stress management workshops, or providing access to external mental health providers, EAPs offer a comprehensive approach to supporting employee mental health.

In conclusion, Employee Assistance Programs are crucial components of public health initiatives in the workplace. By recognizing and addressing the mental health needs of employees, organizations contribute to creating a healthier and more productive workforce. EAPs not only benefit individuals but also have a positive impact on the overall wellbeing of communities. It is essential for employers to invest in these programs to ensure the mental health and wellbeing of their employees.

Chapter 10: Maintaining Mental Health in the Digital Age

The Impact of Technology on Mental Health

In today's digital age, it is impossible to ignore the pervasive influence of technology on our daily lives. From smartphones to social media platforms, technology has revolutionized the way we communicate, work, and entertain ourselves. However, with these advancements come potential consequences, especially when it comes to our mental health.

The rapid rise of technology has created a new set of challenges for individuals and society as a whole. While technology has undoubtedly brought numerous benefits, such as improved access to information and enhanced communication, it has also introduced several negative impacts on mental health.

One of the primary concerns is the constant connectivity that technology provides. We are now more interconnected than ever before, but this has resulted in heightened levels of stress and anxiety. The pressure to be constantly available and responsive can lead to burnout and a sense of overwhelm. Moreover, the addictive nature of technology can lead to compulsive behaviors and a harmful cycle of comparison and self-doubt, as we are constantly exposed to carefully curated versions of others' lives on social media.

Another significant impact of technology on mental health is the decline in face-to-face interactions. As we increasingly rely on digital communication, we lose the valuable social connections and support that come from genuine human interaction. Loneliness and isolation have become prevalent issues in today's society, leading to increased rates of depression and anxiety.

Furthermore, the excessive use of technology has been linked to sleep disturbances and disrupted circadian rhythms. The blue light emitted by screens interferes with our natural sleep patterns, making it harder to fall asleep and stay asleep. This can have detrimental effects on our mental health, as sleep is crucial for cognitive functioning, mood regulation, and overall wellbeing.

While technology has undoubtedly posed challenges to mental health, it is important to note that it can also be a powerful tool for promoting mental wellbeing. Online therapy and mental health apps have made accessing support more convenient and affordable. Additionally, technology can facilitate connections and provide a platform for sharing experiences, reducing the stigma surrounding mental health.

In conclusion, the impact of technology on mental health is a complex and multifaceted issue. While it has brought undeniable benefits, it has also introduced challenges that must be addressed. Striking a balance between utilizing technology for its advantages while minimizing its negative effects is crucial for preserving our mental health and wellbeing in the digital era. By being mindful of our technology use and fostering meaningful connections offline, we can harness the power of technology while protecting our mental health.

Establishing Healthy Technology Habits

In today's fast-paced, technology-driven world, it is essential to establish healthy technology habits to maintain our mental health and overall well-being. The constant use of smartphones, tablets, and computers has become an integral part of our daily lives, but it is important to strike a balance between our digital and offline worlds. This subchapter aims to guide individuals from all walks of life on how to establish healthy technology habits for improved mental health and well-being.

First and foremost, it is crucial to set boundaries with technology usage. Allocate specific times during the day to engage with digital devices and designate technology-free zones, such as the bedroom or dining area. By establishing these boundaries, you can create a healthier relationship with technology and prevent it from encroaching on your personal and social life.

Another vital aspect of healthy technology habits is practicing digital detox. Regularly taking breaks from technology, whether it be for a few hours or an entire day, allows you to recharge and reconnect with the present moment. Engaging in activities such as reading a book, going for a walk, or spending time with loved ones without technology can significantly reduce stress levels and enhance mental well-being.

Additionally, it is important to be mindful of the content we consume online. The internet can be a valuable source of information and connection, but it can also be overwhelming and detrimental to our mental health. Practice discernment and limit exposure to negative or triggering content. Instead, seek out positive and educational resources that uplift and inspire you.

Creating a healthy technology environment is equally crucial. Consider turning off push notifications on your devices to minimize distractions and interruptions. Organize your digital space, decluttering unnecessary apps and files, to promote a sense of calm and order. Moreover, ensure that your screen time is not interfering with your sleep schedule. Establish a technology curfew before bedtime to allow your mind to unwind and prepare for a restful sleep.

By following these guidelines, individuals from all walks of life can establish healthy technology habits that promote mental health and overall well-being. Remember, technology should serve as a tool to enhance our lives, not consume them entirely. With a conscious effort to find balance and set boundaries, we can navigate the digital world more mindfully and thrive in our personal and social lives.

Managing Social Media and Online Presence

In today's digital age, social media has become an integral part of our lives. It has revolutionized the way we connect, communicate, and share information. However, while social media platforms offer great opportunities for public health professionals, they also come with their own set of challenges. This subchapter aims to provide valuable insights and guidance on managing social media and online presence for individuals working in the field of public health.

The Importance of Social Media in Public Health
Social media has the power to amplify public health messages and reach a wide audience. It allows public health professionals to disseminate information quickly, engage with the community, and promote positive health behaviors. By leveraging social media platforms effectively, public health practitioners can raise awareness about important health issues, combat misinformation, and foster a sense of community.

Building a Strong Online Presence
Creating a strong online presence is crucial for public health professionals. It establishes credibility and helps to build trust with the audience. Start by identifying the key platforms where your target audience is active. Develop a clear and consistent brand voice that aligns with your organization's mission and values. Regularly share relevant and reliable content to establish yourself as a thought leader in the field. Engaging with the audience through comments, likes, and shares is vital for building meaningful connections.

Managing Social Media Challenges

While social media offers great opportunities, it is not without its challenges. One of the primary concerns is the spread of misinformation. Public health professionals need to actively combat false information by sharing accurate and evidence-based content. It is also crucial to address any negative comments or feedback promptly and professionally, and to engage in constructive dialogue with the audience.

Ethical Considerations

Public health professionals must adhere to ethical standards when using social media. Respect confidentiality and privacy laws by avoiding sharing personal or sensitive information without proper consent. Be transparent about your affiliations and potential conflicts of interest. Practice cultural sensitivity and avoid engaging in any form of discrimination or harm. Utilize social media responsibly and ensure your actions align with the principles of public health.

Conclusion

Managing social media and online presence is a vital aspect of public health. By leveraging social media platforms effectively, public health professionals can disseminate accurate information, engage with the community, and promote positive health behaviors. However, it is crucial to be mindful of the challenges and ethical considerations associated with social media use. By following best practices and maintaining a strong online presence, public health professionals can make a significant impact on the health and wellbeing of individuals and communities.

Balancing Screen Time and Real-Life Connections

In today's modern world, technology has become an integral part of our daily lives. We are constantly connected to screens, whether it's through our smartphones, tablets, or computers. While these devices have undoubtedly brought numerous benefits, such as increased access to information and enhanced communication, they also come with potential drawbacks. One of the most significant challenges we face is finding a balance between screen time and real-life connections.

Spending excessive time in front of screens can have detrimental effects on our mental health and overall wellbeing. Research has shown that excessive screen time is linked to increased feelings of loneliness, depression, and anxiety. This is because spending too much time in the virtual world can lead to a lack of genuine human connections and meaningful social interactions. It is crucial to recognize the importance of face-to-face interactions and maintain a healthy balance between our digital lives and real-life connections.

To strike this balance, we need to be mindful of our screen time habits and actively make an effort to prioritize real-life connections. Here are some practical tips to help you achieve this balance:

1. Set boundaries: Establish specific periods of the day where you disconnect from screens and engage in activities that promote real-life connections, such as spending time with loved ones, pursuing hobbies, or engaging in physical exercise.

2. Practice active listening: When interacting with others, make a conscious effort to be fully present and actively listen. Put away your devices, maintain eye contact, and show genuine interest in what the

other person is saying. This will strengthen your real-life connections and create a deeper sense of understanding and empathy.

3. Engage in offline activities: Instead of relying solely on digital platforms for entertainment, explore offline activities that foster real-life connections. Join community groups, attend local events, or participate in sports clubs to meet new people and engage in meaningful interactions.

4. Set screen time limits: Utilize screen time monitoring tools or apps that allow you to set limits on your device usage. This will help you become more aware of your screen time habits and encourage you to prioritize real-life connections.

By finding the right balance between screen time and real-life connections, we can enhance our mental health and overall wellbeing. Remember, technology should be a tool that enriches our lives, not an obstacle that hinders genuine human connections. Embrace the healing power of real-life interactions and create a healthier relationship with technology for a more fulfilling and meaningful life.

Chapter 11: Embracing a Holistic Approach to Mental Wellbeing

Integrating Mind, Body, and Spirit

In today's fast-paced world, it is all too easy to get caught up in the chaos and neglect our overall well-being. Our mental health is just as important as our physical health, and it is crucial to find a balance between the two. In this subchapter, we will explore the concept of integrating mind, body, and spirit, and how it can contribute to our overall mental health and well-being.

Integrating mind, body, and spirit is about aligning these three aspects of our being in order to achieve harmony and balance. When we neglect any one of these areas, it can lead to feelings of disconnection, stress, and a decline in our overall mental health. By consciously working on integrating these aspects, we can enhance our physical and mental well-being.

The mind is a powerful tool that can greatly influence our overall health. By practicing mindfulness and engaging in activities such as meditation or journaling, we can calm our minds, reduce stress, and improve our mental clarity. Taking time to reflect on our thoughts and emotions can help us identify any negative patterns or beliefs that may be hindering our well-being.

The body is the vessel through which we experience the world. It is essential to nourish and care for our physical well-being in order to support our mental health. Engaging in regular exercise, eating a balanced diet, and getting enough sleep are all important aspects of maintaining a healthy body. When we take care of our bodies, we not only improve our physical health but also boost our mood and overall mental well-being.

Spirituality is a deeply personal aspect of our being. It can be defined in many ways, depending on individual beliefs and values. Nurturing our spirituality can provide a sense of purpose and meaning in life. Engaging in activities such as prayer, meditation, or spending time in nature can help us connect with our inner selves and find a sense of peace and fulfillment.

Integrating mind, body, and spirit is a lifelong journey that requires mindfulness and self-reflection. By prioritizing our mental health and well-being, we can lead more fulfilling lives and contribute to the overall improvement of public health. So, take a moment today to reflect on how you can integrate mind, body, and spirit in your own life. Remember, the path to healing and well-being starts from within.

Incorporating Alternative Therapies

The field of public health has evolved significantly over the years, recognizing the importance of mental health and wellbeing in overall well-being. As we strive to achieve optimal health, it is crucial to explore various avenues, including alternative therapies, to support our mental and emotional needs.

Alternative therapies encompass a wide range of practices that are not typically considered part of conventional medicine but have shown promising results in improving mental health. These therapies may include acupuncture, yoga, meditation, aromatherapy, and many others.

One of the key benefits of alternative therapies is their holistic approach, treating the individual as a whole rather than focusing solely on symptoms or specific conditions. By addressing the mind, body, and spirit, these therapies aim to restore balance and promote overall well-being.

Acupuncture, for instance, is a traditional Chinese medicine practice that involves the insertion of tiny needles into specific points on the body. It is believed to stimulate the flow of energy, or Qi, and can be beneficial in reducing stress, anxiety, and even managing chronic pain. Many individuals have reported significant improvements in their mental health after incorporating acupuncture into their wellness routine.

Yoga and meditation are other alternative therapies that have gained popularity in recent years. These practices promote mindfulness, connecting the mind and body through movement and breath.

Regular yoga and meditation sessions have been shown to reduce anxiety, improve mood, and enhance overall mental clarity. Additionally, they can boost physical health by improving flexibility, strength, and cardiovascular endurance.

Aromatherapy is another alternative therapy that utilizes essential oils to promote relaxation and emotional well-being. Certain scents, such as lavender and chamomile, are known for their calming properties, while others, like citrus and peppermint, can uplift and energize. Incorporating aromatherapy into your daily routine, whether through diffusers, massage oils, or bath products, can have a profound impact on your mental state and overall sense of well-being.

While alternative therapies should not replace conventional medical treatment, they can serve as valuable complementary tools in managing mental health and promoting overall wellness. It is important, however, to consult with a qualified healthcare professional before incorporating any alternative therapy into your routine, especially if you have pre-existing health conditions or are taking medications.

Incorporating alternative therapies into our daily lives can be a transformative journey towards mental health and well-being. By embracing these holistic practices, we open ourselves up to new possibilities and empower ourselves to take an active role in our own healing journey. Let us explore the world of alternative therapies and discover the immense benefits they can bring to our lives.

Exploring Holistic Practices

In today's fast-paced world, where stress and anxiety have become a part of our daily lives, it is crucial to prioritize our mental health and overall well-being. Traditional approaches to healthcare often focus solely on the physical aspects, neglecting the interconnectedness of our mind, body, and spirit. However, the concept of holistic practices has gained significant attention in recent years, emphasizing the importance of treating the whole person rather than just the symptoms.

This subchapter aims to introduce the audience to the world of holistic practices and their potential benefits for mental health and overall well-being. Whether you are a healthcare professional, a student, a parent, or simply someone seeking to enhance your quality of life, understanding holistic practices can be transformative.

Holistic practices encompass a wide range of approaches, including alternative therapies, mindfulness techniques, and self-care practices. These practices acknowledge that our mental and emotional states are intricately connected to our physical health. By addressing all aspects of our being, holistic practices aim to promote balance, harmony, and optimal well-being.

One of the cornerstones of holistic practices is the incorporation of alternative therapies such as acupuncture, naturopathy, and herbal medicine. These approaches focus on stimulating the body's natural healing mechanisms, promoting physical and mental well-being. By considering the individual as a whole, these therapies offer a personalized approach to healthcare, considering each person's unique needs and circumstances.

Mindfulness techniques, another integral part of holistic practices, involve cultivating awareness, acceptance, and non-judgment in the present moment. These practices, such as meditation, yoga, and deep breathing exercises, can help reduce stress, improve concentration, and enhance overall mental health. By training our minds to be more present and aware, we can gain a deeper understanding of ourselves and develop healthier coping mechanisms.

Self-care practices play a vital role in holistic approaches to well-being. Engaging in activities that nourish our mind, body, and spirit is essential for maintaining optimal mental health. Whether it's engaging in hobbies, spending time in nature, or practicing gratitude, self-care practices remind us to prioritize ourselves and our well-being.

By embracing holistic practices, we can embark on a healing journey that addresses the root causes of mental health issues and promotes overall well-being. This subchapter will provide valuable insight into the different holistic practices available, their potential benefits, as well as practical tips for incorporating them into our daily lives. No matter your background or profession, exploring holistic practices can be a transformative step towards achieving mental health and overall well-being in the fast-paced world we live in.

Finding Balance in Daily Life

In our fast-paced and demanding world, finding balance in daily life has become crucial for our mental health and overall well-being. The constant pressures and responsibilities we face can easily overwhelm us, leaving us feeling stressed, anxious, and exhausted. However, by consciously seeking balance, we can regain control over our lives and cultivate a sense of inner peace.

One of the key aspects to finding balance is prioritizing self-care. Taking care of our physical, emotional, and mental needs should be our top priority. This means making time for exercise, eating nutritious meals, getting enough sleep, and engaging in activities that bring us joy and relaxation. By making self-care a non-negotiable part of our daily routine, we can replenish our energy and better cope with life's challenges.

Another important element in finding balance is setting boundaries. Learning to say no when we feel overwhelmed or when a task doesn't align with our priorities is crucial. We can't please everyone all the time, and it's important to recognize our limits and protect our time and energy. By establishing healthy boundaries, we create space for ourselves and the things that truly matter.

Mindfulness practices play a significant role in finding balance in our daily lives. Taking a few moments each day to engage in mindfulness exercises, such as meditation or deep breathing, can help us manage stress and stay present in the moment. Mindfulness allows us to let go of worries about the past or future, and instead focus on the present, which can greatly reduce anxiety and increase our overall sense of well-being.

Finding balance also involves nurturing our relationships. Connecting with loved ones and building strong support systems is essential for our mental health. Taking the time to cultivate meaningful connections and engage in activities with family and friends can bring us a sense of joy, belonging, and fulfillment.

Lastly, incorporating gratitude into our daily lives can help us find balance. By focusing on what we are grateful for, we shift our perspective and appreciate the positives in our lives. Practicing gratitude regularly can reduce stress, increase resilience, and improve our overall mental health.

In conclusion, finding balance in daily life is essential for our mental health and well-being. By prioritizing self-care, setting boundaries, practicing mindfulness, nurturing relationships, and cultivating gratitude, we can create a harmonious and fulfilling life. Remember, finding balance is a continuous journey, and it's important to be patient and kind to ourselves as we navigate through life's challenges.

Chapter 12: The Journey Towards Mental Health and Wellbeing

Embracing the Healing Journey

In our fast-paced and high-stress modern world, it is more important than ever to prioritize our mental health and wellbeing. The healing journey is a personal and transformative experience that allows us to discover the power within ourselves to achieve mental wellness. This subchapter explores the significance of embracing this journey and how it can positively impact our lives.

In terms of public health, the healing journey holds immense value. Mental health issues have become a global epidemic, affecting people from all walks of life. By embracing the healing journey, we can work towards reducing the stigma surrounding mental health and promoting a more inclusive and supportive society. This subchapter aims to empower every individual to take charge of their own mental health and wellbeing, ultimately contributing to the overall improvement of public health.

The healing journey is not a linear path but rather a process of self-discovery and growth. It begins with acknowledging and accepting the challenges we face, whether they be anxiety, depression, or any other mental health disorder. By embracing these struggles, we open ourselves up to the possibility of healing and transformation.

One crucial aspect of the healing journey is self-care. It is essential to prioritize our physical, emotional, and spiritual well-being. Engaging in activities such as exercise, meditation, and spending time in nature can have a profound impact on our mental health. This subchapter provides practical tips and guidance on incorporating self-care practices into our daily lives, regardless of our busy schedules.

Furthermore, the healing journey entails seeking professional help when needed. Mental health professionals play a vital role in supporting and guiding individuals through their healing process. By encouraging readers to reach out for help, this subchapter aims to break down the barriers that prevent many from seeking the assistance they require.

Ultimately, embracing the healing journey is an act of self-empowerment. It allows us to reclaim our lives, find inner peace, and build resilience. This subchapter emphasizes that the healing journey is not just a means to an end, but a lifelong commitment to self-care and personal growth.

In conclusion, "Embracing the Healing Journey" is a subchapter that addresses the significance of prioritizing mental health and wellbeing in our lives. By embracing this journey, we contribute to the improvement of public health and create a more compassionate and understanding society. This subchapter provides practical guidance on self-care, seeking professional help, and cultivating resilience. It is a call to action for individuals from all backgrounds to embark on their own healing journey and discover the transformative power of mental wellness.

Setting Personal Goals

In our journey towards mental health and wellbeing, setting personal goals plays a crucial role. Goals provide us with direction, purpose, and a sense of accomplishment. They give us something to strive for and help us stay focused on what truly matters to us. Whether you are a student, a working professional, a parent, or anyone else, setting personal goals can greatly contribute to your overall wellbeing.

When it comes to setting personal goals, it is important to be specific and realistic. Vague goals like "be happier" or "get healthier" may not provide the clarity needed to take actionable steps. Instead, break down your goals into smaller, achievable targets. For example, if your goal is to improve your physical health, you could set a specific target of walking for 30 minutes every day or reducing your sugar intake by a certain amount. By setting smaller goals, you can track your progress more effectively and stay motivated along the way.

Another important aspect of setting personal goals is ensuring they are aligned with your values and priorities. Reflect on what truly matters to you and what you want to achieve in different areas of your life, such as career, relationships, health, and personal growth. This will help you set goals that are meaningful to you and increase your chances of success.

It is also beneficial to set both short-term and long-term goals. Short-term goals provide immediate motivation and a sense of accomplishment, while long-term goals keep us focused on the bigger picture. By setting a combination of both, you can experience the satisfaction of achieving smaller milestones while still working towards your larger aspirations.

Furthermore, it is crucial to regularly review and reassess your goals. Life is constantly changing, and what may have been important to you a year ago may no longer hold the same significance today. Take the time to reflect on your progress, adjust your goals if needed, and celebrate your achievements along the way.

Remember, setting personal goals is not about perfection or comparing yourself to others. It is about acknowledging your own desires and aspirations and taking steps towards fulfilling them. By setting personal goals that are specific, aligned with your values, and adaptable, you can embark on a fulfilling journey towards mental health and wellbeing.

Whether you are a student, a working professional, a parent, or anyone else, setting personal goals can greatly contribute to your overall wellbeing. Goals provide us with direction, purpose, and a sense of accomplishment, helping us stay focused on what truly matters. In the realm of public health, setting personal goals is a powerful tool for individuals to take control of their mental health and wellbeing. By encouraging everyone to set personal goals, we can collectively foster a healthier and happier society.

Celebrating Progress and Success

In the journey towards mental health and wellbeing, it is essential to acknowledge and celebrate the progress and successes we achieve along the way. These moments of triumph serve as powerful reminders of our resilience and strength, motivating us to continue our efforts and inspiring others in their own healing journeys.

For individuals working in the field of public health, celebrating progress and success is particularly important. It not only boosts morale and motivation but also provides an opportunity to showcase the positive outcomes achieved through various mental health initiatives. By sharing these success stories, we can inspire others to take action and prioritize their mental health and wellbeing.

One way to celebrate progress and success is by highlighting personal stories of triumph. These narratives serve as powerful testimonials, demonstrating the transformative impact of mental health interventions. By sharing these stories, we can help break the stigma associated with mental health and encourage individuals to seek support without fear or shame.

Furthermore, it is crucial to acknowledge and appreciate the efforts of mental health professionals, researchers, and organizations in driving positive change. Their dedication, expertise, and commitment to improving mental health outcomes deserve recognition. By celebrating their achievements, we can foster a sense of collective pride and encourage further advancements in the field of public health.

Celebrating progress and success should also involve engaging the wider community. Public health initiatives often rely on the participation and support of individuals, communities, and policymakers. By involving them in the celebration, we can foster a sense of ownership and collective responsibility towards mental health and wellbeing. This can be achieved through public events, awareness campaigns, and community engagement programs that highlight the positive impact of mental health interventions.

In conclusion, celebrating progress and success is vital not only for individuals on their healing journeys but also for the field of public health. By sharing personal stories of triumph, recognizing the efforts of mental health professionals, and engaging the wider community, we can inspire others and foster a culture that prioritizes mental health and wellbeing. Let us celebrate every step forward and every success achieved, for they are testaments to the power of resilience and the potential for change.

Sustaining Mental Health and Wellbeing

In today's fast-paced and demanding world, it is crucial for everyone to prioritize their mental health and wellbeing. The journey towards achieving mental health and wellbeing is a lifelong process that requires constant attention and effort. This subchapter of "The Healing Journey: Discovering Mental Health and Wellbeing" aims to provide valuable insights and practical tips on how to sustain and nurture our mental health in order to lead a fulfilling and balanced life.

Public health is a field that is deeply concerned with the health and wellbeing of the population as a whole. Mental health is a significant aspect of public health, as it affects individuals, families, communities, and society as a whole. Therefore, it is essential for public health professionals to understand the importance of sustaining mental health and wellbeing and to promote strategies that support it.

One of the key factors in sustaining mental health and wellbeing is self-care. Self-care involves recognizing and addressing our own physical, emotional, and psychological needs. It means taking time for ourselves, engaging in activities that bring us joy and relaxation, and setting healthy boundaries in our personal and professional lives. By prioritizing self-care, we can recharge our batteries and build resilience to cope with life's challenges.

Another crucial aspect of sustaining mental health and wellbeing is nurturing healthy relationships. Human connection and social support are fundamental to our mental and emotional wellbeing. Building and maintaining positive relationships, whether it's with family, friends, or colleagues, can provide a sense of belonging, understanding, and validation. It is important to invest time and effort into cultivating these connections, as they can serve as a source of strength and support during difficult times.

In addition to self-care and healthy relationships, maintaining a balanced lifestyle is essential for sustaining mental health and wellbeing. This includes adopting healthy habits such as regular exercise, a balanced diet, and sufficient sleep. Physical health and mental health are closely intertwined, and by taking care of our bodies, we can also support our emotional and psychological wellbeing.

Finally, seeking professional help when needed is an important aspect of sustaining mental health and wellbeing. There is no shame in reaching out for support from mental health professionals, as they are trained to provide guidance and assistance in navigating life's challenges. It is important to remember that seeking help is a sign of strength, not weakness.

In conclusion, sustaining mental health and wellbeing is a vital aspect of living a fulfilling and balanced life. By practicing self-care, nurturing healthy relationships, maintaining a balanced lifestyle, and seeking professional help when needed, we can promote our own mental health and contribute to the wellbeing of our communities. Public health professionals play a crucial role in raising awareness about the importance of mental health and implementing strategies to support it. Together, we can create a society that values and prioritizes mental health and wellbeing for everyone.

Conclusion: A Lifetime of Mental Health and Wellbeing

In this journey through the pages of "The Healing Journey: Discovering Mental Health and Wellbeing," we have embarked on a quest to understand the intricacies of our minds, emotions, and the importance of mental health. Now, as we reach the end of this enlightening book, we must reflect on the valuable lessons we have learned and how they can positively impact our lives.

Mental health is not an isolated experience; it is an essential component of our overall wellbeing. It is a lifelong journey that requires our constant attention and care. By focusing on our mental health, we can develop resilience, enhance our relationships, and achieve personal growth. The knowledge gained from this book empowers us to take charge of our mental health and make informed choices for a happier and more fulfilling life.

For each and every one of us, mental health should be a priority. It is not a luxury reserved for a few, but a fundamental right for all. Public health plays a crucial role in ensuring that mental health services are accessible and affordable to everyone, regardless of their socio-economic background. By advocating for mental health policies and increased funding, we can create a society that prioritizes the mental wellbeing of its citizens.

One of the key takeaways from this book is the recognition that mental health is not a destination but a continuous journey. It requires ongoing self-reflection, self-care, and a willingness to seek help when needed. We have learned various strategies and techniques to nurture our mental wellbeing, such as practicing mindfulness, engaging in physical activity, and fostering meaningful connections with others.

The importance of destigmatizing mental health cannot be emphasized enough. By openly discussing our mental health struggles, we break down barriers and create a supportive environment for everyone. Let us remember that seeking help is a sign of strength, not weakness. Together, we can eliminate the shame and silence surrounding mental health issues and build a society that embraces and supports each individual's journey towards wellness.

As we conclude our exploration of mental health and wellbeing, let us carry the knowledge gained from this book into our daily lives. This is not the end but the beginning of a lifelong commitment to our mental health. By prioritizing self-care, seeking support when needed, and advocating for better mental health services, we can create a brighter future for ourselves and future generations.

May this book serve as a guiding light on your journey towards mental health and wellbeing. Remember, you are not alone in this endeavor. Together, we can create a world where mental health is a top priority, and every individual can thrive and flourish.

www.ingramcontent.com/pod-product-compliance
Lightning Source LLC
LaVergne TN
LVHW012046070526
838201LV00079B/3637